Black Women and da 'Rona

THE FEMINIST WIRE BOOKS
Connecting Feminisms, Race, and Social Justice

SERIES EDITORS

Monica J. Casper, Tamura A. Lomax, and Darnell L. Moore

EDITORIAL BOARD

Brittney Cooper, Aimee Cox, Keri Day, Suzanne Dovi, Stephanie Gilmore, Kiese Laymon, David J. Leonard, Heidi R. Lewis, Nakisha Lewis, Adela C. Licona, Jeffrey Q. McCune Jr., Joseph Osmundson, Aishah Shahidah Simmons, Stephanie Troutman, Heather M. Turcotte

ALSO IN THE FEMINIST WIRE BOOKS

Lavender Fields: Black Women Experiencing Fear, Agency, and Hope in the Time of COVID-19, edited by Julia S. Jordan-Zachery

A Love Letter to This Bridge Called My Back, edited by gloria j. wilson, Joni B. Acuff, and Amelia M. Kraehe

Black Girl Magic Beyond the Hashtag: Twenty-First-Century Acts of Self-Definition, edited by Julia S. Jordan-Zachery and Duchess Harris

The Chicana Motherwork Anthology, edited by Cecilia Caballero, Yvette Martinez-Vu, Judith C. Pérez-Torres, Michelle Téllez, and Christine Vega

Them Goon Rules: Fugitive Essays on Radical Black Feminism, by Marquis Bey

BLACK WOMEN and DA 'RONA

Community, Consciousness, and Ethics of Care

EDITED BY **JULIA S. JORDAN-ZACHERY**
AND **SHAMARA WYLLIE ALHASSAN**

THE UNIVERSITY OF
ARIZONA PRESS

TUCSON

The University of Arizona Press
www.uapress.arizona.edu

We respectfully acknowledge the University of Arizona is on the land and territories of
Indigenous peoples. Today, Arizona is home to twenty-two federally recognized tribes, with
Tucson being home to the O'odham and the Yaqui. Committed to diversity and inclusion, the
University strives to build sustainable relationships with sovereign Native Nations and Indig-
enous communities through education offerings, partnerships, and community service.

ISBN-13: 978-0-8165-4853-8 (paperback)
ISBN-13: 978-0-8165-4963-4 (ebook)

Cover design by Leigh McDonald
Cover art: *Generations* by Jemma Morris / LouLou Art Studio
Typeset by Sara Thaxton in 10.25/15 Minion Pro with Millimetre and Helvetica LT Std

Library of Congress Cataloging-in-Publication Data
Names: Jordan-Zachery, Julia S., 1971– editor. | Alhassan, Shamara Wyllie, 1986– editor.
Title: Black women and da 'Rona : community, consciousness, and ethics of care / edited by
    Julia S. Jordan-Zachery and Shamara Wyllie Alhassan.
Other titles: Feminist wire books.
Description: Tucson : University of Arizona Press, 2023. | Series: The feminist wire books |
    Includes bibliographical references and index.
Identifiers: LCCN 2022029955 (print) | LCCN 2022029956 (ebook) | ISBN 9780816548538
    (paperback) | ISBN 9780816549634 (ebook)
Subjects: LCSH: Women, Black—Social conditions—21st century. | Women caregivers—
    Social conditions. | Feminism and racism. | COVID-19 (Disease)—Social aspects.
Classification: LCC HQ1163 .B536 2023 (print) | LCC HQ1163 (ebook) | DDC 305.48/896—
    dc23/eng/20220712
LC record available at https://lccn.loc.gov/2022029955
LC ebook record available at https://lccn.loc.gov/2022029956

To all Black femmes, girls, and women we lost to COVID-19, to those who are living with long COVID, and to all who have lost loved ones, we dedicate this collection to you—may you be protected always.

CONTENTS

FOREWORD

Keisha L. Bentley-Edwards

In one of my favorite books, Zora Neale Hurston's *Their Eyes Were Watching God*, the lead character, Janie, is slapped and then hugged by her grandmother (Nanny) when, as a teenager, she is found enjoying the company and touch of a man. Nanny's slap is meant to wake Janie up to the realities of Black womanhood, while the embrace acknowledges the unfairness of these realities. Nanny then tells Janie,

Honey, de white man is de ruler of everything as fur as Ah been able tuh find out. Maybe it's some place way off in de ocean where de black man is in power, but we don't know nothin' but what we see. So de white man throw down de load and tell de nigger man tuh pick it up. He pick it up because he have to, but he don't tote it. He hand it to his womenfolks. De nigger woman is de mule uh de world so fur as Ah can see. Ah been prayin' fuh it tuh be different wid you. Lawd, Lawd, Lawd! (Hurston [1937] 2005, 62)

This scene of gendered racial socialization has always resonated with me. Colloquially called "The Talk," racial socialization includes the implicit and explicit messages that youth receive about what to expect from society, what society expects from them, and how to safely navigate these issues as a Black person. Gendered racial socialization consists of the messages that address the intersecting identities of race and gender, in this case of a Black girl burgeoning into her womanness. Through direct conversations and modeling behaviors, contemporary socialization messages indicate the expectation of Black women's unbounded strength and Black Girl Magic—essentially, making a way out of no way. Black women are still tasked with saving our families, nations, and spirits before tending to our own needs and desires. The distinctive nature of the "ride or die" Black woman is evident in that there is no comparable ubiquitous phrase for Black men. Black women are not only expected to bear the weight of other people's decisions but to do so with flair and grace.

In 2020, the COVID-19 pandemic spread globally, highlighting systemic health, social, and economic racial disparities. Black American women disproportionately faced care responsibilities for children and elders, despite making sixty-three cents for every white man's dollar (Childers, Hegewisch, and Mefferd 2021; Laster Pirtle and Wright 2021). In the first half of 2020, three high-profile, state-sanctioned murders of Black people occurred in the United States, including the murder of Breonna Taylor, a Black woman. By summer, Black women and queer people were leaders in one of the largest global protest movements against state violence toward Black people (Blain 2020), while simultaneously facing disproportionate COVID-19 morbidity and mortality. By the fall of 2020, a presidential election was underway in which the incumbent campaigned using racist tropes against Black people, Latinxs, Muslims, people with disabilities, immigrants, and any other group that misaligned with nostalgic racism and prejudice. Again, Black women were moved to canvas, campaign, and cosign for the Democratic Party for victory at the presidential and legislative levels (Dolan, Deckman, and Swers 2022)—while continuing to face disproportionate COVID-19 death and disability. In 2020, Black women delivered. By the end of 2020, Black women's voices were gathering to say that carrying these burdens with very little reward was not sustainable.

Drs. Julia S. Jordan-Zachery and Shamara Wyllie Alhassan, the editors of *Black Women and da 'Rona: Community, Consciousness, and Ethics of Care*, could see how Black women would be employed as the mules of the world during the pandemic. What is unique about this collection is that it also serves as a guide to the other part of Nanny's statement, where life could or would be *different* for our children and ourselves. So this book is not only about centering the real-time experiences and perspectives of Black women throughout the pandemic but also about centering the care, concern, grief, and joy of Black women. In *Black Women and da 'Rona*, the diverse viewpoints of Black women from throughout the Diaspora are bridged together to recognize common and divergent outlooks on what happened in the pandemic, as they experienced it. Although this book is about this significant and global moment in time, the COVID-19 pandemic is about more than the 'Rona. Who faces the greatest harms and who gains the greatest profits from the pandemic-related disruptions to everyday life depends on whose well-being is prioritized and whose well-being is sacrificed. Black women's narratives in the moment demonstrate that the concerns that have been amplified during the COVID-19 pandemic extend beyond the virus itself and are revealed in our experiences in the tech industry, the media, sexual exploration, politics, and simply growing into our womanhood. These issues will endure beyond the containment of COVID-19. What tools do we, as Black women, need in order to be heard, seen, and valued? How can the expectations put on our lives by society be *different*? Ultimately, that is the array of realism in conversation with hope that can be found in *Black Women and da 'Rona*.

Dr. Jordan-Zachery talks about how the ancestors nudged and then prodded her until she moved forward with this project. I am thankful that she listened to them, as you, the reader, will soon agree. As a scholar who studies racism and gender discrimination, the pandemic has elevated interest in my own work. This increased interest has tasked me with explaining the nuances of racism while simultaneously experiencing personal and collective racism, while grieving, and while caretaking. There would be moments when I would hear the whispers of my mother and grandmother, my own ancestors: "You can't pour from an empty cup." Although these whispers would remind me to ease how much I poured into others, they didn't give me sufficient guidance on how I could center my needs and actually stop pouring into people who should have known better. *Black Women and da 'Rona* tells the story of Black women at their most stretched, and how we can still pour into each other while also replenishing our cups (spirits).

Through Nanny, our ancestor Zora Neale Hurston warned us how Black women were the mules of the world—*Black Women and da 'Rona* shows us that Black women are #MulesNoMore.

Bibliography

Blain, Keisha N. 2020. "Black Women Are Leading the Movement to End Police Violence." *Washington Post*, October 1, 2020. https://www.washingtonpost.com/outlook/2020/10/01/black-women-are-leading-movement-end-police-violence/.

Childers, Chandra, Ariane Hegewisch, and Eve Mefferd. 2021. *Shortchanged and Underpaid: Black Women and the Pay Gap*. Washington, D.C.: Institute for Women's Policy Research, July 2021. https://iwpr.org/iwpr-publications/fact-sheet/shortchanged-and-underpaid-black-women-and-the-pay-gap.

Dolan, Julie, Melissa M. Deckman, and Michele L. Swers. 2022. *Women and Politics: Paths to Power and Political Influence*. Lanham, MD: Rowman and Littlefield.

Hurston, Zora Neale. (1937) 2005. *Their Eyes Were Watching God*. Philadelphia: J. B. Lippincott Company. Reprint, New York: HarperCollins. Citations refer to the HarperCollins edition.

Laster Pirtle, Whitney N., and Tashelle Wright. 2021. "Structural Gendered Racism Revealed in Pandemic Times: Intersectional Approaches to Understanding Race and Gender Health Inequities in COVID-19." *Gender and Society* 35, no. 2: 168–79. https://doi.org/10.1177/08912432211001302.

ACKNOWLEDGMENTS

This collection would not be possible had it not been for the ancestors who gently spoke to Julia about putting together this volume—we thank you for your wisdom. We thank you, the contributors, who wrote alongside COVID as they fought to save their lives. And we thank Kristen Buckles and the entire editorial team at the University of Arizona Press and the Feminist Wire for your careful engagement.

Black Women and Da 'Rona

We Will Not Be Disappeared

Black Women's Responses to COVID-19

Julia S. Jordan-Zachery and Shamara Wyllie Alhassan

During the summer of 2020, in the midst of the COVID-19 pandemic, the ancestors visited Julia and offered her this project. While she initially resisted, the ancestors, in their divine wisdom, were patient in their way of knowing. Ancestral knowledge recognizes the value of the "speaking center" (hooks 1989, 15). The "speaking center" affords Black women the opportunity to speak of their lived experiences as they become the "subject," thereby being "transformed in consciousness and being" (15). But as hooks warns us, "To speak as an act of resistance is quite different from ordinary talk, or the personal confession that has no relation to coming into political awareness, to developing critical consciousness" (14). This work is intentionally and critically curated in a manner that centers the voices of Black women (and *Black* is used not to collapse differences, but as a way of embracing African-descended women and African women) to help us critique power and also to imagine a different way of being in the midst of the calls to go back to "normal" in a COVID world. *Black Women and da 'Rona* is about care, community, and consciousness that centers the lived realities of Black women. To understand Black women's experiences with COVID-19, we have to dip into the past, allowing the past to meet the present so that we can enter into the future with radical care. Thus, while the essays may be situated in the present moment of COVID-19, we encourage you all to read in a manner that suspends time as we tend to record it and imagine time the way that Black women have had to as part of their survival practices.

Black women with a particular type of consciousness probably raised their eyebrows at the claim that COVID-19 was the "great equalizer" or at the notion that "we're all in this together." It is not that Black women are cynical; it is that we operate from rememory (to borrow from Toni Morrison 1987) and hauntology (to borrow from Viviane Saleh-Hanna 2015). COVID-19 is a relatively new pandemic, but Black women are haunted. They are haunted by the pandemics of the past, and the rememory is enough to know that this iteration is not some great equalizer and that we are not all in this together. History tells us a different story, and it is a story that we will not soon forget.

We, Black women, have been living in pandemics stretching as far back as colonialism and enslavement. We have been impacted by pandemics, including the 1918–19 Spanish flu and the HIV and AIDS pandemic that began in the 1980s and persists today. COVID-19, like HIV and AIDS, has once again revealed the precarious existence of Black women—those on the continent of Africa and those who constitute the African Diaspora. What COVID-19 also shows is how Black women can be disappeared from the histories of pandemics. In the initial stages of the HIV/AIDS pandemic, Black women were also disappeared (Jordan-Zachery 2017 and Berger 2004). The annals of the often compared Spanish flu reveal how Black women's stories and experiences have been disappeared or are treated in a limited manner at best. Indeed, what we have on record shows an eerie similarity between the 1918–19 and COVID-19 pandemics.

Consider the following:

"This pesky flu's all over town! And white and black and rich and poor are all included in its tour."

COVID-19 infection and mortality glaringly confirm for us the profound nature of the social de-

When the 1918 influenza epidemic began its deadly tour across the United States, African Americans were already beset by a host of major public health, medical, and social problems that shaped how they experienced the epidemic and how the epidemic affected them. By 1918, medical and public health reports had documented that African Americans suffered higher morbidity and mortality rates than white people for several diseases. (Gamble 2010, 114)

terminants of health (SDOH). In essence, these social and demographic characteristics describe the intersectionality of economics, education, employment, and environment on human health. Research indicates that the SDOH, defined as the environments where people play, work, and live, account for up to 80% of health risk (Singh et al. 2017). The racial/ethnic disparities of COVID-19 illuminate for us how social and economic inequities have real and often dire health consequences. For Black Americans, the SDOH are further undergirded by the prevailing lived experience of systemic US racism contributing to the recurring health inequities experienced during global pandemics. (Williams 2020, 441)

While, to some extent, the impact of these pandemics on Black communities and the centering of how the pandemics are mapped onto previously existing inequalities have been documented, we argue that the voices of Black women are generally absent. As was the case for both the Spanish flu and COVID-19 pandemics, data is not disaggregated along lines that allow us to speak explicitly to those that are raced and gendered (alongside other identity markers) in specific ways. We know what the data say as it relates to race or gender, but never race and gender simultaneously.

We offer this edited volume to recognize the politics and processes that often lead to Black women not being seen and remembered. *Black Women and da 'Rona: Community, Consciousness, and Ethics of Care* is not the complete telling of how Black women experience and live with multiple pandemics—COVID-19 and the ongoing state-sanctioned violence that leaves us dead both physically and spiritually—but it is a necessary component of what we hope will become a tapestry of Black women telling their tales. We use the concept of fugitive breath and anti-Black gendered COVID-19 necropolitics as one way of situating Black women's multidimensional experiences.

A Sisters of the Yam Fugitive Breath Poetics

My breath is prayer, the shape of life, evolving name. All I can see is just the blur that says life moves. I stay in prayer, and reach to listen for your breath.

—Alexis Pauline Gumbs, *Undrowned*

Ancestral knowledge is the oxygen fueling our blood flow and expanding our lungs. We learn from deep breathing and listening within and beyond our species. COVID-19 came to transform our intimacies and break many of us from our care circles through its vicious snatching of breath. But as Alexis Pauline Gumbs reminds us, "Breathing in unbreathable circumstances is what we do every day in the chokehold of racial gendered ableist capitalism" (2020, 4). Expanding our meditations on breathing, Gumbs allows us to consider the ways that marine mammals, trees, plants, and other living beings share in our collective ability to breathe. The stories embraced here are our offering of shared breath—a guide to reclaiming our lungs, to drawing upon our foremothers, and to enacting our mothers' lessons about how to keep breathing and insist on life during COVID. Our book is written as a collective inhale and exhale for Black women because we know that the ways we are thinking and feeling and how we are living and thriving through these unbreathable conditions is the key to shape-shifting practices that create new futures rooted in the expansive science fiction of our being (brown 2019). Just as some marine mammals must learn how to breathe in water upon their birth, so can we harness our ancestral and present knowledges to chart impossible futures. Nannie Helen Burroughs reminded us in 1909 that as Black women, "We specialize in the wholly impossible" (quoted in Berry and Gross 2020, 1). As a statement of futurity out of the precipice of anti-Blackness, Black women's excessive possibility is always beyond the realm of reason imposed by social norms and mores. Across geographies, time, and space as we encounter COVID-19 and face present challenges, Gumbs reminds us, we are flexible, durable, and expansive enough to learn "to breathe in ways [we] haven't breathed before. To learn [our] blood in ways [we] didn't know it" (39). In this time, we must use ancestral knowledge flowing through our blood to learn new ways of collective breath, because even as we are forced into isolation, we realize that our physical distance does not overdetermine our social connection, our care work, and our collective healing, which necessitates our intimacy.

When the ancestors called Julia to initiate this project, she set up small care circles between authors to encourage and foster writing in community. She created an ethic of care contract to protect the authors and enable a sort of intimacy that perhaps was not thought possible in virtual spaces but allowed authors to grow through the relationships they formed. When Julia invited me, Shamara, to join in her care work as a co-editor of this volume and as an author, she encouraged me to take the latitude and elasticity to write, edit, and commune with authors in ways that honored our aliveness, both personal and collective. Through this work, we built an editorial model based on bell hooks's Sisters of the Yam. Sisters of the Yam was a support group hooks formed in the 1990s after reading Toni Cade Bambara's *The Salt Eaters* with a class she was teaching. hooks was inspired by a character in Bambara's work who asked, "Are you sure sweetheart, that you want to be well?" (quoted in hooks [1994] 2015, 6). "Only an affirmative response makes healing possible," hooks responded (6). Beginning here, hooks created a support group with other Black women who wanted to be well and find ways of healing pain. hooks writes, "Black female self-recovery, like all Black self-recovery, is an expression of a liberatory political practice. Living as we do in a white-supremacist capitalist patriarchal context that can best exploit us when we lack a firm grounding in self and identity (knowledge of who we are and where we have come from), choosing 'wellness' is an act of political resistance" (7). bell hooks passed on December 15, 2021, just a couple of weeks before we completed this introduction. Still, her work and her meditations on collective healing guided both Julia and me as we cultivated this work. When we think of the intimacy that hooks taught us to nurture in our healing work and that Julia's ancestral knowledge allowed her the visionary presence to create in this edited volume, we begin to respond to a question Gumbs poses when she asks, "What are the scales of intimacy and the actual practices that would teach us how to care for each other beyond obligation or imaginary duties?" (2020, 86). In thinking of the scales of our intimacy during COVID, we need not journey farther than our breath, which necessitates our individual and collective wellness. As we think with Gumbs and hooks, it is clear that our breathing is inherently fugitive in that it relies on our connectivity, our intimacy, our planetary wellness, our aliveness in the face of the anti-Black gendered COVID-19 necropolitics. We realize that through our ancestral and editorial practice, we can create a sisters of the yam fugitive breath poetics that shapes our thinking about the ways Black women have created community in the midst of an impossible COVID reality.

When we think of Black women and girls breathing, we think of our aliveness (Quashie 2021). We think of the "feeling/knowledge" that makes sense of our realities and the poetics that allows us to share

this knowing with others (Christian 1987, 72). In this moment of adversity, we harness our writerly traditions to remember the strategies
our mothers employed to make a way out of no way. Barbara Christian and Audre Lorde remind us of the importance of our breathing
on the page. Christian writes, "I can only speak for myself. But what
I write and how I write is done to save my own life. And I mean that
literally" (77). Audre Lorde reminds us of the necessity of our poetics
that writing helps us to share: "We can train ourselves to respect our
feelings and to transpose them into a language so they can be shared.
And where that language does not yet exist, it is our poetry which
helps to fashion it" (1984, 25–26).

Our breathing on the page allows us to language the sensual nature
of pushing air through lips slightly open and inhaling air through
nostrils slightly flared. Our writing together created a fugitive breath
poetics that allowed us to find aliveness even in the interstitial space of
COVID. COVID necessitated that we learned to breathe with a mask
covering those parts of ourselves that are normally left free. Writing in
COVID taught us to share airspace with others through the constric-
tions of quarantine. Our sisters of the yam editorial praxis allowed
us to acknowledge the pain of forced labor for capitalism, which en-
dangers our lives and puts our families at risk for wages that barely
allow us to subsist. Through a series of foreclosures that can only be
understood through the lens of anti-Black gendered COVID-19 necropolitics, Black women's capacity for inventing strategies of mutual
aid, finding pleasure in the most precarious places, and focusing on
breathing on the page as we form a poetics that speaks to our aliveness
are some of the ways we resisted, balanced, and theorized our place
through COVID.

Drawing from Achille Mbembe's notion of necropolitics, which he
defines as "contemporary forms of subjugation of life to the power of
death" (quoted in Smith 2016, 32), Christen Smith develops the notion of anti-Black gendered necropolitics to recognize the ways that

Black women are impacted by state violence, both by being targets and through the sequelae, or afterlife, of state violence that causes enduring trauma for families. As Shamara meditated upon our present reality, she developed the term *anti-Black gendered COVID-19 necropolitics*, which uses Smith's concept of anti-Black gendered necropolitics to provide a portal for understanding this moment so that we can move beyond statistical quantification of people dying and foreground the strategies of aliveness innovated by Black women thinking about the trauma of COVID and its afterlife.

Smith writes, "I use sequelae (in its plural form) here to describe the gendered, reverberating, deadly effects of state terror that infect the affective communities of the dead" (2016, 31). *Sequelae* is a medical term used to describe the enduring impacts of illness on patients even after a disease is cured—for example, as Smith discusses, psychologists have used *sequelae* to describe post-traumatic stress disorder in war veterans. Smith examines how the traumatic loss of children or parents at the whim of the state causes durable and lasting adverse health outcomes that resemble PTSD. The concept of sequelae, she argues, allows people to grasp the enduring adversity that cannot be quantified and is often not public.

During the summer of 2020, at the height of the COVID pandemic and after the successive murders of unarmed Black people, including Breonna Taylor, George Floyd, and Ahmaud Arbery, the largest racial uprising in U.S. history organized to proclaim that Black Lives Matter (Buchanan, Bui, and Patel 2020). Created by three Black women, Alicia Garza, Patrisse Cullors, and Ayọ Tometi (formerly known as Opal Tometi), the notion of Black Lives Matter was a simple, commonsense affirmation that met the moment of despair by proclaiming that Black people are valuable. While this statement became an affront to anti-Black necropolitical logics, this phrase also became a poetics that allowed people to translate their experiences of the world into a reality that resonated across social identities, geographies, and quarantine. All of this occurred because organizers dared to talk back to the state, share breath while chanting "no justice, no peace," and use their bodies to stop traffic and physically interrupt business as usual. Black women's rebellious practice of sustaining Black life and loving themselves and each other, whether virtually or in person, provided radical portals for developing an ethic of care that undoes the sequelae of COVID and anti-Black gendered necropolitics.

Since the first cases of COVID, physical sequelae of the virus, or long COVID, has been identified by the Centers for Disease Control and Prevention (CDC) in the United States as lingering health issues related to never fully recovering from the virus. Research and data collection concerning the etiology of long COVID is ongoing as more information about the virus becomes available. But there is not much data about how many Black women are impacted by long-COVID symptoms. Medical studies suggest that COVID disproportionately impacts women and that Black people are also disproportionately impacted. While there is emergent data on the ways that people who are Black *and* women are impacted, a full accounting remains elusive (Walton, Campbell, and Blakey 2021). As medical professionals, public health officials, and epidemiologists continue to study the health impacts of COVID-19 on Black populations, this inquiry can be augmented by attention to Smith's discussion of anti-Black gendered necropolitics and Black women's choices to be well. We contend that, as part of assessing the enduring legacy of the pandemic, the physical sequelae of COVID-19 must be studied with attention to the broader enduring trauma of families directly impacted by the loss of loved ones.

This moment of concentrated energy provides portals for rethinking the way we relate to one another, the way we share, and the way we care for one another. Called in by the pressing need to heal and restore, we witnessed and participated in making space for restorative and planetary justice, which will ultimately build equitable relationships where communion among all living beings is supported and our planet is sustained. This rethinking was amplified by calls for the abolition of policing and prisons, reimagining safety, a focus on healing, and renewed commitment to realizing freedom in this lifetime. COVID-19 forced many of us to remain inside and to relate to each other through masks, gloves, hand sanitizer, and Zoom calls. Our relationships were reimagined as we were made aware of the imminence of our physical mortality. But amid this forced distancing, people in turn created force fields for justice in massive protests where thousands of people gathered outside to make embodied calls for justice. Their demands for justice allowed epidemiologists to understand the virus better because they discovered that open air and masks prevented the super spread of viral infection (Ramjug 2020). As we reflect upon this delicate moment and all of the many unknowns of the safety of our relations, our breath is made fugitive by the conditions that inform our ability to exist. Still, we are ever reminded that our breath is also our guide to our shared poetics. It is the way to healing through unfreedom, our way of insisting on life and aliveness in the face of impossibility. As Gumbs writes, "Are you still breathing? This is an offering towards our evolution, towards the possibility that instead of continuing the trajectory of slavery, entrapment, separation, and domination and making our atmosphere unbreathable, we might instead practice another way to breathe" (2020, 4). As Black women forming a sisters of the yam fugitive breath poetics through editorial intention and authorial affirmation, we affirm what Nannie Helen Burroughs knew at the turn of the twentieth century: "We specialize in the wholly impossible."

Holding Our Breath as We Breathe: The Impact of COVID-19 on Black Women

In light of anti-Black gendered COVID-19 necropolitics and fugitive breath poetics, to say that Black women exist in fragile spaces is not an overstatement. Before COVID, data showed us the generational and lifelong challenges Black women often faced. During COVID, these challenges have not lessened; in fact, they are exacerbated. Post-COVID, if we are to imagine a world with Black women, we need to confront these fragile spaces and design alternatives that allow Black women and their communities to flourish. As a result of race-gender oppressions, Black women face housing, health, and income inequities, among others.

COVID is simply now mapped onto these historical and long-standing inequities, thus giving way to race-gender necropolitics. The challenge of analyzing the impact of COVID-19 on Black women, especially across geographical locations, is that data is not systematically collected. In the United States, Johns Hopkins University, early in the pandemic, established the Coronavirus Resource Center. This digital platform offers both a global map and a more specific U.S. map to track COVID-19-related cases and deaths. As of June 17, 2022, there were 3.9 million cases of COVID and 101,880 deaths in South Africa, 66,300 cases and 1,262 deaths in Guyana, and 82,643 cases and 478 deaths in Barbados (Coronavirus Resource Center 2020a); the United States has reported over 86 million cases and over 1 million deaths (2020b). The United Nations (UN) also offers comprehensive global data on COVID-19 cases and resulting deaths. A systemic problem is that the data does not offer within-group analysis, and data is not collected in a systematic manner that lends to comparisons. Thus, we know that in the United States, 1 in 289 Black Americans died (Gawthrop 2021) and over 384,000 women died (Centers for Diseases Control and Prevention n.d.). We have no data on how many Black women were infected and died due to the virus. This is a challenge globally. For all the conversation on disparate impacts and the recognition that viruses impact communities differently depending on social location, in 2022, with a global pandemic, society is not collecting data that recognizes that some of us are simultaneously Black and women. One would have thought that the HIV/AIDS pandemic would have informed how data is collected, and we would do differently as we face COVID-19.

COVID-19, as is the case with HIV and AIDS, is having a disparate impact on Black women, and this is true across geographical locations. While we may not know the cases and deaths of Black women specifically, there is enough data that allows us to map the impact of this virus on the lives of Black women. The impact is both direct and indirect; it is financial and emotional, physical and psychological. The impact of COVID-19 seems all-encompassing, and in the following pages, we try to offer a glimpse into how this virus has impacted Black women thus far—and we recognize that COVID-19 is rapidly changing and evolving. For example, as we write about the impact on Black women, the world is being introduced to new strains of the virus. So the nature of this pandemic is fluid. Given its fluid nature, we offer data on several variables, treating them in a discrete manner while realizing that this is not a linear impact, doing our best to represent what Black women may be experiencing.

We recognize that COVID-19 is not singularly responsible for the impacts faced by Black girls and women but instead is mapped onto what existed prior to the spread of the virus. First, we present data on maternal and child health. From there, we offer a snapshot on the virus's financial impact, followed by the impacts on mental health, housing insecurity, intimate partner violence, and other violences. We ask what the impact is on differently abled Black women and transgender women. We do this as we NEED to have our story recorded in history so that we are not vanished in the way that Black women vanished in the recording of the Spanish Flu of 1918–19.

We wish we could say that the story we are about to tell is uplifting. It is not. Simply put, Black women who were in peril prior to COVID-19 are now facing even more challenges. Now we ask, "Who will hear Black women?"

Maternal Health

What do we know from the past? According to Stein, Ward, and Cantelmo (2020),

> During the Ebola epidemic in West Africa in 2014–2016, the use of
> reproductive and maternal healthcare services plummeted so much
> that maternal and neonatal deaths and stillbirths indirectly caused by
> the epidemic outnumbered direct Ebola-related deaths. . . . Some of
> these women stopped going to facilities due to fear of infection and in-
> creased physical and financial barriers. Others were denied care if they
> were suspected of having Ebola as many facilities were not equipped to
> provide maternal healthcare to infected women.

COVID is resulting in similar patterns, with women being particularly nervous and hesitant to seek medical care (Gordon 2021; Goyal
et al. 2021).

In Latin America and the Caribbean, women and children are facing extreme health conditions, which may result in declines in any
health progress they have made over the years. In other words, women
and children are facing a regression in their health. Therefore, we can
anticipate increases in maternal mortality, for example (Castro 2020);
indeed, Black women in the United Kingdom are five times as likely
as their white counterparts to experience a pregnancy-related death
(Reuters 2020), and in the United States, they are three to four times
as likely to die (National Partnership for Women and Families 2018).
In Brazil, Black-identified women face disproportionate pregnancy
and postpartum challenges (de Souza Santos et al. 2020).

"COVID-19 exacerbates the issues around Black maternal health,"
said Marcela Howell, president of In Our Own Voice: National Black
Women's Reproductive Justice Agenda, in 2020 (quoted in Whaley
2020). The challenges faced by pregnant women are multifaceted. For

example, increased food insecurity can result in malnutrition and micronutrient deficiencies, which can harm not only the woman but also the fetus. Consequently, both mother and fetus can face increased risk of infection and death. Pregnant women who are low income and lower resourced also face the challenge of accessing quality care (a challenge that existed prior to COVID-19 and is now worsened). Women are experiencing limited availability to essential health care services, and in some cases, women are giving birth without their partners or even a companion (Bobrow 2020). COVID has also impacted reproductive care in general, and as such, some women are experiencing limited access to abortion and birth control as a result of both logistical challenges and ongoing political threats that limit access (Connor et al. 2020).

Financial Impact

Stagnant wages, underemployment, and poverty have all been part of Black women's experiences before COVID-19. Black women have not all had the same economic experience resulting from the downturn in the economy, and we recognize that some Black women, such as the editors of this volume, have been able to benefit from their jobs and the attending financial security, and they have been able to shelter in place while working. While it is important to recognize that Black women are not monolithic, we concentrate on those who have been disproportionately impacted. We believe that we are only as strong as we can be when all of us can freely pursue a safe and secure life. Black women are disproportionately economically poor.

Data tells us that Black workers (and Indigenous and Hispanic workers), relative to white workers, face greater and increasing economic insecurity from COVID-19. According to Gould and Wilson, "There are three main groups of workers in the COVID-19 economy: those who have lost their jobs and face economic insecurity, those who are classified as essential workers and face health insecurity as a result, and those who are able to continue working from the safety of their homes" (2020, 4). Overwhelmingly, Black women are not in the third category of workers. In the United States, Black women find themselves categorized as "essential" and "frontline" workers. This has translated into them and their families facing extreme risk. According to the National Women's Law Center, more than one in three Black-identified women in the United States serve as essential workers in frontline jobs. These women are working as sales personnel, nursing assistants, health-care workers, and domestic care workers, for example. It is also estimated that many of these women are immigrants (Neely 2020). Given their place in the employment sector, many of these women have no safety net to buffer them from unemployment and have limited or no access to health care.

Mental Health

The overall well-being of Black women tends to be precarious even in "normal" times. Much of this precarity manifests in terms of "stress" and other mental health issues and is a result, in part, of the race-gender-class oppression many Black women face. This precarity persists during COVID. Consider that "Black pregnant women reported a greater likelihood of having their employment negatively impacted, more concerns about a lasting economic burden, and more worries about their prenatal care, birth experience, and post-natal needs" (Gur et al. 2020). Black pregnant women are stressed. Connor et al. tell us that "multifactorial stress is uniquely exacerbated among women during Covid-19" (2020). Additionally, Black communities tend to have lower access to mental health and substance-abuse care. This has been worsened by the stay-at-home orders. Their frontline status, schooling children from home, and financial and housing instability, in conjunction with the continued assaults on Black bodies, contributes to the high level of stress faced by Black women during COVID (University of Michigan School of Public Health 2020).

Housing Insecurity

By all accounts, COVID has worsened housing insecurity for those already at the edge of finding and maintaining stable housing. A Center for American Progress report reveals, "Before COVID-19, half of all renters were moderately or severely cost-burdened, with at least 30 to 50 percent of their household income going toward housing costs. Cost-burdened renters, particularly those of color, are the most at risk of eviction due to the increased likelihood of missing rent payments. People of color, who have faced higher rates of lost employment during the pandemic, continue to be disproportionately cost-burdened and at increased risk of eviction" (Lake 2020). Before the pandemic, Black women were disproportionately exposed to evictions (Desmond 2014), and this has only worsened during the pandemic given the economic insecurity they face.

In response to economic insecurity caused by the pandemic recession, the U.S. federal government issued an eviction moratorium as part of the 2020 Coronavirus Aid, Relief, and Economic Security (CARES) Act. This moratorium prohibited landlords from filing new evictions in federally supported or financed housing. Initially, the moratorium was set to expire in July of 2020; it was extended through July 2021. While it prevented eviction, it did not recuse tenants from paying any portion of their late rent. Thus, Black women who benefited from the mortarium now have to find a way of paying their rent or face eviction. What we know is that Black women are experiencing severe economic insecurity. A CNN headline read, "The US Economy Lost 140,000 Jobs in December. All of Them Were Held by Women" (Kurtz 2021). Another headline, in *The Cut*, declared, "COVID Is Pushing Black Mothers Out of the Workforce at a Staggering Rate" (Aggeler 2020). In Canada, Black women are experiencing the highest unemployment rates of any demographic (Gordon 2020), and so it is anticipated that they will face a similar situation as Black women in the United States. Many African nations are also facing increasing housing instability. According to a report issued by UN-Habitat, "Risks of housing eviction due to lack of income and consequential rent arrears are . . . high. In Africa, the share of people renting their accommodation can be as high as 70% in urban areas" (2020, 10). Black women, regardless of geographical location, are in perilous situations regarding housing. Many of us need affordable housing and are constantly facing being unhoused, and COVID has worsened this reality.

Intimate Partner Violence and Other Violences

Black women experience multiple forms of violence. The UN reports that prior to the pandemic, "243 million women and girls, aged 15–49 experienced sexual and/or physical violence by an intimate partner in the past year." The report goes on to say that since the onset of the pandemic, "domestic violence has intensified" (UN n.d.). While the conditions that expose women to intimate partner violence (IPV) are the same regardless of the pandemic, the pandemic has exacerbated women's exposure to this violence.

Researchers have highlighted a number of factors that influence Black women's exposure to IPV. It is suggested that Black women's overexposure to structural violence, racism, sexism, poverty, and lack of access to health care contributes to their disproportionate experience with IPV (Hampton, Oliver, and Magarian 2003; Oliver 1989). Beth Richie (1996, 2012), among others, centers identity, race, gender, class, etc., as factors that influence how Black women not only experience IPV but how they are treated by law enforcement. Stereotypes, such as the emasculating Black woman, are also thought to shape

Black women's experiences with IPV (Bell and Mattis 2000; Bent-Goodley 2005, 2007; Gillum 2009; West 2004).

In the United States, Black women accounted for 30 percent of all IPV-related deaths among all women between 2003 and 2014 (Petrosky et al., 2017). Non-white women in the United Kingdom also face disproportionate impacts of IPV (Femi-Ajao 2018). Women in Nigeria (Benebo, Schumann, and Vaezghasemi 2018) and Jamaica (Turner-Jones 2020) are also facing high rates of IPV.

Often framed as the pandemic within the pandemic, Black women's experiences with IPV have been exacerbated during COVID-19. Many women now find themselves sheltering in place, with limited financial resources due to the economic downturn, socially isolated with their abusers, and limited access to public spaces. As Tamara Y. Jeffries writes, "It's a formula that puts sisters at an even greater risk of physical, emotional, or financial abuse" (2020).

Differently Abled, Incarcerated, and Transgender Black Women

There is much ado about Black women's exposure to COVID-19. Some of us are engaging in conversations that bring us to a post-pandemic period and how we begin to build infrastructure to support Black women. However, in the midst of these conversations, some bodies are missing. Differently abled, incarcerated, and transgender Black women are shadow bodies (Jordan-Zachery 2017) in the public discourses on COVID-19. Their absence is in part due to how data is collected; we collect data on race or gender, ignoring that some are simultaneously raced and gendered. Some bodies go missing partly because of boundaries (Cohen 1999) and who is allowed into public discourses as the result of policing who is considered "normal" and respectable.

"Black people with disabilities are in a health equity crisis in the United States that is compounded by the COVID-19 pandemic—we just don't know exactly how bad it is" (Young 2020). Young is not exaggerating when he claims that we simply do not know how differently abled Black individuals, and differently abled Black women specifically, are experiencing COVID-19. Black feminists speak of invisibility and the need to bring Black women from the margin to the center. If there was ever a need for us to systematically apply this, it is now. One in four Black-identified individuals are living with a disability (Courtney-Long et al. 2017). Research tells us that this population is challenged in terms of securing employment (Mitra and Kruse 2016) and accessing health care (Campbell et al. 2009) and affordable housing. We can ill afford to not pay attention, socially and politically, to how differently abled Black women are experiencing and living with COVID-19. Thus, we need to expand the boundaries to make space for the needs of differently abled Black women.

And it is the same case for incarcerated Black women. Black girls are more than three times as likely as white girls to be locked up, and Black women are almost twice as likely to be incarcerated relative to their white counterparts (Sentencing Project 2020). In an interview with Nick Charles (2020), Donna Hylton (a previously incarcerated prison activist) stated, "These populations are medically compromised long before incarceration. We didn't have resources before incarceration; imagine the communities inside prisons and jails." Incarcerated Black women experience limited testing and medical resources, and social distancing is not available. Consequently, by May 14, 2020, "Black inmates encompassed 60 percent of COVID-19 deaths in New York's prison system, even though they were around 50 percent of the state's incarcerated population" (ACLU West Virginia 2020). We need to discuss how this population, incarcerated Black girls and women, are disappearing and or in danger of disappearing right before our eyes as they become ill and/or die in prisons and jails.

In the shadow of our public discourse are Black transgender women and how they are living with COVID-19. According to the *2015 U.S.*

Transgender Survey (James, Brown, and Wilson 2017), Black transgender people face the most severe economic and housing effects among LGBTQ+ communities. The same survey tells the story of their overexposure to violence, homelessness, and poverty, and limited access to shelters, health care, and the labor market (James, Brown, and Wilson 2017). The Black LGBTQ+ population faces a number of structural risk factors as described above, and many experience isolation from families, thus heightening their vulnerability to COVID-19. At the time of this writing, there was no data that spoke to how many Black transgender individuals were impacted by COVID-19, or how. Consequently, the story of this group is relatively sparse, not because we do not want to tell the story but because there is limited data that allows us to tell the story.

Black women, regardless of geographical or social location, find themselves occupying COVID-19 forward-facing spaces. The story told here is limited as data was not always readily available, and such data is concentrated in certain countries. But this is what we know:

- There is a feminization of care work, and much of that care work is being carried out by poor women, immigrants, and women of color.
- Stay-at-home orders exacerbate gender violence.
- Black women have to provide care across multiple fronts—in and outside of their homes.
- Black women face economic, housing, and job insecurity.
- Black women disproportionately work as essential frontline workers and therefore play critical roles in the political economy.
- Black women's access to quality health care is compromised by racism.
- Black women are stressed.
- COVID-19 maps onto existing structures of oppression.

Some might refer to Black women as "heroes" and "strong." This can result in Black women not being seen, and as such, the full impact of the virus on our lives can go underreported and not responded to via public policies. Black women can ill afford to be rendered invisible—we are the canaries in the coal mine, showing all that is broken in society. As societies attempt to manage COVID-19 and imagine a post-COVID life, we need to hear Black women.

The Stories of Black Women and da 'Rona: An Overview of the Book

Included in the following pages are nine chapters that span African and African Diasporic women's experiences with COVID-19. The essays in this volume speak to anti-Black gendered COVID-19 necropolitics, singularly and collectively, and call on us to grapple with (1) how Black women are talking back to COVID-19 and also state-sanctioned violence; (2) how Black women engage in care, a type of care that extends beyond "self-care" to protect themselves and their communities; and (3) how Black women's agency and actions can shape equitable and just policies.

Addressing, in part, this notion of survival is chapter 1, "'Cyah Leave We Alone, We Rel Stayin' Home': A Black Caribbean Diasporic Reflection on Healing Through Movement, Creating Home, and Time-Warping During COVID-19." Sherine Andreine Powerful and Onisha Etkins, using their experiences as members of the Black Caribbean Diaspora, explore how they rely on healing and pleasure during and beyond the COVID-19 pandemic. What they present is a "documented application and reclamation of Black Caribbean people's agency in sustaining our ability to survive and flourish in the face of oppression and existential threats." Endia Hayes, in "*Femme Mixing*: On an Erotics of Slowness and Its Wet Futures," chapter 2, relies on the creative work of Megan Thee Stallion to show how Black women bend time, thereby creating space for them to be seen and heard. Hayes states, "Using the erotics of slowness prominent in 2020 *femme mixing*, I attend to how Black women and femmes express, and listen to, the gatherings of our innermost selves as sound and time drags. Meaning, as we believe that our fluctuations from crying to anger, from relief to sitting in the dark binging Netflix or social media, have felt lonely, we have in fact never been alone. Rather, forced isolation was just an uncovering of an erotic life under slowness." Here we have a reimagining of slowness as a means of entering the erotic, as understood by Audre Lorde, which allows Black women to assert their identity even in oppressive spaces.

The following chapters bring us deeper into structural and systemic responses to COVID-19 for our immediate and future times. In chapter 3, "Black Women and Coronavirus in the United Kingdom: The Need for a Black Feminist Epidemiology," Jenny Douglas looks at how Black women in the United Kingdom are experiencing COVID-19. Douglas explores the "need to develop opportunities for Black women to lead research to develop epidemiological approaches and methodologies based on a Black feminist epistemology so that we can fully record, investigate, analyze, and understand the impact of COVID-19 on Black women," and argues that a Black feminist perspective is beneficial for understanding not just the epidemiology but also the public narratives that can influence policy decisions. Chapter 4, "*Wanawake Wavumilivu*: Tanzanian Women's Voices of Survivance" by Amber Walker and Rhonda M. Gonzales, utilizes the narratives of Black women and girls from three Tanzanian locations and territories, living in different villages, to tell their stories of agency, fear, hope, and community survival. This essay illuminates how the COVID-19 pandemic has affected their ability to be in and with the community and how it is affecting the livelihood of these Black women in Tanzania and the work they are doing to survive. In chapter 5, "Exploring Resiliency and

Coping Strategies Among Black Women Enrolled in Graduate School During COVID-19 and Overlapping Racial Injustices," Breauna Marie Spencer, Sharnnia Artis, Nitya Mehrotra, Marjorie Shavers, and Stacie LeSure analyze institutional failures and their impacts on Black graduate students. Using the lived experiences of Black women graduate students, they show how institutions perpetually fail to support their needs and articulate institutional practices that are designed to see and hear Black women simultaneously.

Chapter 6, "Da 'Rona and a Virtual Kitchen Table Politics of Community" by Ashley E. Hollingshead and Michelle Meggs, shows how "the creation of online communities as kitchen table gathering spaces falls within and extends this trajectory toward recognition of Black people's subjectivity and humanity." According to Hollingshead and Meggs, the kitchen table, virtual or in real life, is a transformative space and in this era of COVID-19 provides Black women an opportunity to engage in purposeful action as we shelter in place. Candace S. Brown, Kaja Dunn, Kendra Jason, Janaka B. Lewis, and Tehia Starker Glass's chapter 7, "Black Motherschooling: Creating a Liberatory Community for Home Education," shows how Black women professors respond to Black death by reaffirming the lives of their children. Such action is taking place alongside these women, also breathing into their own lives as they now have to school from home. Through vignettes, the authors detail how motherschooling is deeply entrenched in Black feminist practices, as, indeed, "at the heart of motherschooling is resistance, liberation, and joy." Furthermore, "Motherschooling allows our Black children to navigate fear and anxiety. It prepares them for how the world may treat them and gives context to what they see on the morning news. It allows Black children to build healthy relationships with others. It nurtures Black boys and girls as they are, on their own terms." The authors offer not just a praxis of motherschooling but also suggest how such acts can impact educational policy.

Chapter 8, Breauna Marie Spencer's "The Narratives of Black Women Techies: An In-Depth Qualitative Investigation of the Experiences of Black Women in Tech Organizations During the COVID-19 Pandemic," asks us to consider how Black women in the tech industry manage racial-gender battle fatigue. Relying on qualitative interviews of Black women with varied experiences in the tech industry, Spencer brings to the forefront how stay-at-home orders have actually worked to shield Black women from race-gender oppression. According to Spencer, "The onliness that Black women are required to experience due to their Blackness and womanhood causes them to question their sense of belonging in predominately white work environments and presents challenges to their overall well-being," and they have found some relief from not interacting with their colleagues on a daily basis. While this is not a long-term solution to racism and sexism, it begs the question of how organizations can, in general, protect Black women and not just through rhetoric.

The final chapter by Shamara Wyllie Alhassan offers us a way of closing the volume by focusing on those who joined the ancestral realm and asks us to meditate on our breathing as a guide for our mourning and remembering ourselves by insisting that we will survive. Entitled "Fugitive Breath, Breathing Bones: Ancestral Guide for Abolishing Anti-Black Gendered COVID-19 Necropolitics," this essay recognizes that too many of us are uttering "I can't breathe" as our last words before we transition from the physical realm to the elsewhere. While our living becomes prelude to death, how does sitting with death and still breathing become a fugitive act, a radical praxis that insists upon our living? To this end, this essay continues to honor the ancestors we have gained by recommitting our breathing in the service of reparation and justice. Patrisse Cullors, a cofounder of the Black Lives Matter movement, states that the Black Lives Matter movement is "a spiritual movement. . . . Part of our calling as people who do this work for Black lives is to lift our people up, both in their living, but also in their death. . . . The need to lift our folks up feels so incredibly spirit-driven for me. . . . It is literally almost resurrecting a spirit so they can work through us to get the work that we need to get done" (Molina 2020). Black Lives Matter as a spiritual affirmation, a speaking in of life, a giving of breath; a fugitive mourning in anti-Black space is our offering to honor our ancestors who continue to work through us. Closing with our breath as living tribute to all those who have transitioned to become our ancestors, all those living with the enduring sickness of COVID-19, and the families moving through trauma, we offer our breathing as a framework for engaging in collective mourning, collective joy, and healing to activate life-giving futures.

Recognizing the politics and processes that often lead to Black women not being seen and remembered, we offer this edited volume, *Black Women and da 'Rona: Community, Consciousness, and Ethics of Care*, as a tapestry of Black women telling their own tales and warping time as they inhale and exhale, holding on to the preciousness of breath. The essays in this volume speak to how Black women theorize their experiences of COVID-19 and, in turn, shape our understandings of the epidemiology of COVID-19, using cases studies based on their experiences in England, living in-between spaces in the Caribbean, women's health in Tanzania, the sonic sound of Black women's wetness and slowness, and "motherschooling" in the southern United States. From these perspectives, Black women write themselves beyond statistical calculations of sickness and death. Black women write beyond the perpetual destruction and suffering of life under anti-Black gendered COVID-19 necropolitics and into the slow sensuousness of our bodies, the joy that comes with dancing and cooking, and the virtual kitchen table and the futures that we know hold space for us. Black women write about a world reshaped and made new by a pandemic that destroyed much but revealed much more about the conditions Black women have discussed, proclaimed, and lived. COVID-19 is a portal for a new world (Roy 2020). In these pages, Black women help this world materialize through their insistence on challenging the necropolitical guarantee of death and insisting on life. Black women's conversations about life shift the geography of reason to feature the tensions, complexities, and joys that come through living in relationships with others, perhaps physically distant but socially close. Breathe!

Bibliography

ACLU West Virginia. 2020. "Racial Disparities in Jails and Prisons: COVID-19's Impact on the Black Community." June 12, 2020. https://www.acluwv
.org/en/news/racial-disparities-jails-and-prisons-covid-19s-impact-black
-community.

Aggeler, Madeline. 2020. "COVID Is Pushing Black Mothers Out of the Workforce at a Staggering Rate." *The Cut*, November 12, 2020. https://www.thecut
.com/2020/11/black-mothers-pushed-out-of-workforce-at-staggering-rate
-covid.html.

Bell, Carl C., and Jacqueline Mattis. 2000. "The Importance of Cultural Competence in Ministering to African American Victims of Domestic Violence." *Violence Against Women* 6, no. 5 (May): 515–32. https://doi.org/10.1177/1077
8010022182001.

Benebo, Faith Owunari, Barbara Schumann, and Masoud Vaezghasemi. 2018. "Intimate Partner Violence Against Women in Nigeria: A Multilevel Study Investigating the Effect of Women's Status and Community Norms." *BMC Women's Health* 18 (August): 136. https://doi.org/10.1186/s12905-018-0628-7.

Bent-Goodley, Tricia B. 2005. "Culture and Domestic Violence: Transforming Knowledge Development." *Journal of Interpersonal Violence* 20, no. 2 (February): 195–203. https://doi.org/10.1177/0886260504269050.

———. 2007. "Health Disparities and Violence Against Women: Why and How Cultural and Societal Influences Matter." *Trauma, Violence, and Abuse* 8, no. 2 (April): 90–104. https://doi.org/10.1177/1524838007301160.

Berger, Michele. 2004. *Workable Sisterhood: The Political Journey of Stigmatized Women with HIV/AIDS*. Princeton, NJ: Princeton University Press.

Berry, Daina Ramey, and Kali Nicole Gross. 2020. *A Black Women's History of the United States*. Boston: Beacon Press.

Bobrow, Emily. 2020. "A Chaotic Week for Pregnant Women in New York City." *New Yorker*, April 1, 2020. https://www.newyorker.com/science/medical
-dispatch/a-chaotic-week-for-pregnant-women-in-new-york-city.

brown, adrienne marie. 2019. *Pleasure Activism: The Politics of Feeling Good.* Chico, CA: AK Press.

Buchanan, Larry, Quoctrung Bui, and Jugal K. Patel. 2020. "Black Lives Matter May Be the Largest Movement in U.S. History." *New York Times,* July 3, 2020. https://www.nytimes.com/interactive/2020/07/03/us/george-floyd-protests-crowd-size.html.

Campbell, Vincent A., Jamylle A. Gilyard, Lisa Sinclair, Tom Sternberg, and June I. Kailes. 2009. "Preparing for and Responding to Pandemic Influenza: Implications for People with Disabilities." *American Journal of Public Health* 99, no. S2 (October): S294–300. https://doi.org/10.2105/AJPH.2009.162677.

Castro, Arachu. 2020. *Challenges Posed by the COVID-19 Pandemic in the Health of Women, Children, and Adolescents in Latin America and the Caribbean.* Panama City, Panama: UNICEF and the United Nations Development Programme, September 2020. https://www.unicef.org/lac/en/reports/challenges-posed-covid-19-pandemic-health-women-children-and-adolescents.

Centers for Disease Control and Prevention. n.d. COVID Data Tracker. "Demographic Trends of COVID-19 Cases and Deaths in the US Reported to CDC." Updated June 15, 2022. https://covid.cdc.gov/covid-data-tracker/#demographics.

Charles, Nick. 2020. "Black Female Inmates and COVID-19: Medically Compromised, Vulnerable and Neglected." NBC News, April 11, 2020. https://www.nbcnews.com/news/nbcblk/black-female-inmates-covid-19-medically-compromised-vulnerable-neglected-n1189086.

Christian, Barbara. 1987. "The Race for Theory." *Cultural Critique,* no. 6 (Spring): 51–63. https://doi.org/10.2307/1354255.

Cohen, Cathy. 1999. *The Boundaries of Blackness: AIDS and the Breakdown of Black Politics.* Chicago: University of Chicago Press.

Connor, Jade, Sarina Madhavan, Mugdha Mokashi, Hanna Amanuel, Natasha R. Johnson, Lydia E. Pace, and Deborah Bartz. 2020. "Health Risks and Outcomes That Disproportionately Affect Women During the COVID-19 Pandemic: A Review." *Social Science and Medicine* 266 (December): 113364. https://doi.org/10.1016/j.socscimed.2020.113364.

Coronavirus Resource Center. 2020a. "Global Map." Updated June 17, 2022. https://coronavirus.jhu.edu.

———. 2020b. "U.S. Map." Updated June 17, 2022. https://coronavirus.jhu.edu.

Courtney-Long, Elizabeth A., Sebastian D. Romano, Dianna D. Carroll, and Michael H. Fox. 2017. "Socioeconomic Factors at the Intersection of Race and Ethnicity Influencing Health Risks for People with Disabilities." *Journal*

of Racial and Ethnic Health Disparities 4 (April): 213. https://doi.org/10.1007
/s40615-016-0220-5.

Desmond, Matthew. 2014. *Poor Black Women Are Evicted at Alarming Rates,
Setting Off a Chain of Hardship.* How Housing Matters Policy Research Brief.
Chicago: MacArthur Foundation, March 2014. https://www.macfound.org
/media/files/hhm_research_brief_-_poor_black_women_are_evicted_at
_alarming_rates.pdf.

de Souza Santos, Debora, Mariane de Oliveira Menezes, Carla Betina Andreucci,
Marcos Nakamura-Pereira, Roxana Knobel, Leila Katz, Heloisa de Oliveira
Salgado, Melania Maria Ramos de Amorim, and Maira L. S. Takemoto.
2020. "Disproportionate Impact of Coronavirus Disease-19 (COVID-19)
Among Pregnant and Postpartum Black Women in Brazil Through Structural Racism Lens." *Clinical Infectious Diseases* 72, no. 11 (June): 2068–69.
https://doi.org/10.1093/cid/ciaa1066.

Femi-Ajao, Omolade. 2018. "Intimate Partner Violence and Abuse Against
Nigerian Women Resident in England, UK: A Cross-Sectional Qualitative
Study." *BMC Women's Health* 18: 1–13, e123. https://doi.org/10.1186/s12905
-018-0610-4.

Gamble, Vanessa N. 2010. "'There Wasn't a Lot of Comforts in Those Days':
African Americans, Public Health, and the 1918 Influenza Epidemic." *Public
Health Reports (Washington, D.C.: 1974)* 125, supplement 3: 114–22. https://
doi.org/10.1177/00333549101250S314.

Gawthrop, Elisabeth. 2021. "The Color of Coronavirus: COVID-19 Deaths by
Race and Ethnicity in the U.S." APM Research Lab, updated June 16, 2022.
https://www.apmresearchlab.org/covid/deaths-by-race.

Gillum, Tameka L. 2009. "Improving Services to African American Survivors
of IPV." *Violence Against Women* 15, no. 1 (January): 57–80. https://doi.org
/10.1177/1077801208328375.

Gordon, Deb. 2021. "Women Not Getting the Healthcare They Need During
Covid-19, New Survey Shows." *Forbes*, March 26, 2021. https://www.forbes
.com/sites/debgordon/2021/03/26/women-not-getting-the-healthcare-they
-need-during-covid-19-new-survey-shows/?sh=720626a64d0a.

Gordon, Julie. 2020. "Black, Minority Women in Canada Left Behind in COVID-19
Job Recovery." Reuters, December 15, 2020. https://www.reuters.com/article/us
-health-coronavirus-canada-employment/black-minority-women-in-canada
-left-behind-in-covid-19-job-recovery-idUSKBN28P2O2.

Gould, Elise, and Valerie Wilson. 2020. *Black Workers Face Two of the Most
Lethal Preexisting Conditions for Coronavirus—Racism and Economic In-*

equality. Washington, D.C.: Economic Policy Institute, June 1, 2020. https://www.epi.org/publication/black-workers-covid/.

Goyal, Manu, Pratibha Singh, Kuldeep Singh, Shashank Shekhar, Neha Agrawal, and Sanjeev Misra. 2021. "The Effect of the COVID-19 Pandemic on Maternal Health Due to Delay in Seeking Health Care: Experience from a Tertiary Center." *International Journal of Gynecology and Obstetrics* 152, no. 2 (October): 231–35. https://doi.org/10.1002/ijgo.13457.

Gumbs, Alexis Pauline. 2020. *Undrowned: Black Feminist Lessons from Marine Mammals*. Chico, CA: AK Press.

Gur, Raquel E., Lauren K. White, Rebecca Waller, Ran Barzilay, Tyler M. Moore, Sara Kornfield, Wanjiku F. Njoroge, et al. 2020. "The Disproportionate Burden of the COVID-19 Pandemic Among Pregnant Black Women." *Psychiatry Research* 293 (November): 113475. https://doi.org/10.1016/j.psychres.2020.113475.

Hampton, Robert, William Oliver, and Lucia Magarian. 2003. "Domestic Violence in the African American Community: An Analysis of Social and Structural Factors." *Violence and Victims* 9, no. 5 (May): 522–57. https://doi.org/10.1177/1077801202250450.

hooks, bell. 1989. *Talking Back: Thinking Feminist, Thinking Black*. Boston: South End Press.

———. (1994) 2015. *Sisters of the Yam: Black Women and Self-Recovery*. Boston: South End Press. Reprint, New York: Routledge. Citations refer to the Routledge edition.

James, Sandy E., Carter Brown, and Isaiah Wilson. 2017. *2015 U.S. Transgender Survey: Report on the Experiences of Black Respondents*. Washington, D.C., and Dallas, TX: National Center for Transgender Equality, Black Trans Advocacy, and National Black Justice Coalition, September 2017. https://www.transequality.org/sites/default/files/docs/usts/USTS-Black-Respondents-Report.pdf.

Jeffries, Tamara Y. 2020. "For Black Women Suffering Domestic Abuse, Coronavirus Quarantines Are Life Threatening." *Essence*, December 6, 2020. https://www.essence.com/news/domestic-violence-coronavirus/.

Jordan-Zachery, Julia S. 2017. *Shadow Bodies: Black Women, Ideology, Representation, and Politics*. New Brunswick, NJ: Rutgers University Press.

Kurtz, Annalyn. 2021. "The US Economy Lost 140,000 Jobs in December. All of Them Were Held by Women." CNN Business, January 8, 2021. https://www.cnn.com/2021/01/08/economy/women-job-losses-pandemic/index.html.

Lake, Jaboa. 2020. *The Pandemic Has Exacerbated Housing Instability for Renters of Color*. Washington, D.C.: Center for American Progress, October 30,

2020. https://www.americanprogress.org/issues/poverty/reports/2020/10/30 /492606/pandemic-exacerbated-housing-instability-renters-color/.

Lorde, Audre. 1984. "Poetry Is Not a Luxury." In *Sister Outsider: Essays and Speeches*, 25–27. Crossing Press Feminist Series. Trumansburg, NY: Crossing Press.

Molina, Alejandra. 2020. "Black Lives Matter Is 'a Spiritual Movement,' Says Co-Founder Patrisse Cullors." Religion News Service, June 15, 2020. https:// religionnews.com/2020/06/15/why-black-lives-matter-is-a-spiritual-move ment-says-blm-co-founder-patrisse-cullors/.

Morrison, Toni. 1987. *Beloved*. New York: Penguin.

Mitra, Sophie, and Douglas Kruse. 2016. "Are Workers with Disabilities More Likely to Be Displaced?" *International Journal of Human Resource Man-agement* 27, no. 14: 1550–79. https://doi.org/10.1080/09585192.2015.1137616.

National Partnership for Women and Families. 2018. *Black Women's Maternal Health*. Washington, D.C.: National Partnership for Women and Families, April 2018. https://www.nationalpartnership.org/our-work/health/reports /black-womens-maternal-health.html.

National Women's Law Center. 2020. "Wage Gap Deepens the Economic In-security of Black Women Workers on Front Lines of the Pandemic, New NWLC Analysis Reveals." August 13, 2020. https://nwlc.org/press-releases /wage-gap-deepens-the-economic-insecurity-of-black-women-workers-on -front-lines-of-the-pandemic-new-nwlc-analysis-reveals/.

Neely, Megan Tobias. 2020. "Essential and Expendable: Gendered Labor in the Coronavirus Crisis." The Clayman Institute for Gender Research, June 3, 2020. https://gender.stanford.edu/news-publications/gender-news/essential -and-expendable-gendered-labor-coronavirus-crisis.

Obaji Jr., Philip. 2020. "Nigeria's #EndSARS Protesters Draw Inspiration from Black Lives Matter Movement." *USA Today*, October 26, 2020. https://www .usatoday.com/story/news/world/2020/10/26/nigerias-endsars-protesters -draw-inspiration-black-lives-matter/6044452002/.

Oliver, W. 1989. "Sexual Conquest and Patterns of Black-on-Black Violence: A Structural-Cultural Perspective." *Violence and Victims* 4, no. 4 (Winter): 257–71. https://pubmed.ncbi.nlm.nih.gov/2487138/.

Petrosky, Emiko, Janet M. Blair, Carter J. Betz, Katherine A. Fowler, Shane P. D. Jack, and Bridget H. Lyons. 2017. "Racial and Ethnic Differences in Homi-cides of Adult Women and the Role of Intimate Partner Violence—United States, 2003–2014." *Morbidity and Mortality Weekly Report (MMWR)* 66, no. 28 (July): 741–46. http://dx.doi.org/10.15585/mmwr.mm6628al.

Quashie, Kevin Everod. 2021. *Black Aliveness, Or A Poetics of Being*. Durham, NC: Duke University Press.

Ramjug, Peter. 2020. "Racial Justice Protests Were Not a Major Cause of COVID-19 Infection Surges, New National Study Suggests." News@Northeastern, August 11, 2020. https://news.northeastern.edu/2020/08/11/racial-justice-protests-were-not-a-major-cause-of-covid-19-infection-surges-new-national-study-finds/.

Reuters. 2020. "UK Tackles Higher Maternal Mortality Rates for Black Mothers." Reuters, September 15, 2020. https://www.reuters.com/article/uk-britain-health-mothers/uk-tackles-higher-maternal-mortality-rates-for-black-mothers-idUSKBN25T1KM.

Richie, Beth E. 1996. *Compelled to Crime: The Gender Entrapment of Battered Black Women*. New York: Routledge.

——. 2012. *Arrested Justice: Black Women, Violence, and America's Prison Nation*. New York: New York University Press.

Roy, Arundhati. 2020. "The Pandemic Is a Portal." *Financial Times*, April 3, 2020. https://www.ft.com/content/10d8f5e8-74eb-11ea-95fe-fcd274e920ca.

Saleh-Hanna, Viviane. 2015. "Black Feminist Hauntology: Rememory the Ghosts of Abolition?" *Champ pénal* 12 (March). https://doi.org/10.4000/champpenal.9168.

Scarry, Elaine. 1985. *The Body in Pain: The Making and Unmaking of the World*. New York: Oxford University Press.

Sentencing Project. 2020. *Incarcerated Women and Girls*. Washington, D.C.: Sentencing Project, updated May 2022. https://www.sentencingproject.org/publications/incarcerated-women-and-girls/.

Smith, Christen. 2016. "Facing the Dragon: Black Mothering, Sequelae, and Gendered Necropolitics in the Americas." *Transforming Anthropology* 24, no. 1 (April): 31–48. https://doi.org/10.1111/traa.12055.

Stein, Dorit, Kevin Ward, and Catherine Cantelmo. 2020. "Estimating the Potential Impact of COVID-19 on Mothers and Newborns in Low- and Middle-Income Countries." *Medium*, April 15, 2020. https://healthpolicyplus.medium.com/estimating-the-potential-impact-of-covid-19-on-mothers-and-newborns-in-low-and-middle-income-3a7887e4a0ff.

Turner-Jones, Therese. 2020. "Putting a Stop to Domestic Violence." *Jamaica Observer*, February 16, 2020. http://www.jamaicaobserver.com/editorial/putting-a-stop-to-domestic-violence_187120?profile=1097.

UN (United Nations). n.d. "How COVID-19 Impacts Women and Girls." Accessed June 17, 2022. https://interactive.unwomen.org/multimedia/explainer/covid19/en/index.html.

UN-Habitat. 2020. *COVID-19 in African Cities: Impacts, Responses and Policies*. Nairobi, Kenya: UN-Habitat, June 2020. https://unhabitat.org/sites/default/files/2020/06/covid-19_in_african_cities_impacts_responses_and_policies_2.pdf.

University of Michigan School of Public Health. 2020. "Surviving the Coronavirus While Black: Pandemic's Heavy Toll on African American Mental Health." University of Michigan School of Public Health, May 2020. https://sph.umich.edu/news/2020posts/pandemics-toll-on-african-american-mental-health.html.

Walton, Quenette L., Rosalyn Denise Campbell, and Joan M. Blakey. 2021. "Black Women and COVID-19: The Need for Targeted Mental Health Research and Practice." *Qualitative Social Work* 20, no. 1–2: 247–55. https://doi.org/10.1177%2F1473325020973349.

West, Carolyn M. 2004. "Black Women and Intimate Partner Violence: New Directions for Research." *Journal of Interpersonal Violence* 19, no. 12 (December): 1487–93. https://doi.org/10.1177%2F0886260504269700.

Whaley, Natelegé. 2020. "Black Maternal Health Week Highlights COVID-19's Impact on Black Pregnancy." *Supermajority*, April 14, 2020. https://supermajority.com/2020/04/black-maternal-health-week-highlights-covid-19s-impact-on-black-pregnancy/.

Williams, Lovoria, B. 2020. "COVID-19 Disparity Among Black Americans: A Call to Action for Nurse Scientists." *Research in Nursing and Health* 43, no. 5 (July): 440–41. https://doi.org/10.1002/nur.22056.

Winston, Ali. 2020. "Prosecutors Are Using Gang Laws to Criminalize Protest." *The Appeal*, September 1, 2020. https://theappeal.org/gang-laws-criminalize-protest/.

Young, Daniel. 2020. "Black, Disabled, and Uncounted." National Health Law Program, August 7, 2020. https://healthlaw.org/black-disabled-and-uncounted/.

CHAPTER I

"Cyah Leave We Alone, We Rel Stayin' Home"

A Black Caribbean Diasporic Reflection on Healing Through Movement, Creating Home, and Time-Warping During COVID-19

Sherine Andreine Powerful and Onisha Etkins

Imagine you've just entered the fete you've been looking forward to all week. The selector[1] warms up with some calypso, the food and libations beckon from the side table, and early birds like you and your crew border the party's perimeter, eyes closed and bodies swaying as they anticipate the crescendo of guests and music. Time passes, slow and swift, mirrored by the music's steady progression to middle school dancehall,[2] and you open your eyes to see the crowd thickening as the speakers' bass deepens. You move closer to the center and join strangers who are now your dancing partners. There is such lightness, such freeness, such liveliness to the movements of your arms, your waist, your legs. Next thing you know, you're drenched and out of breath, but enlivened by the vibes and mellowed by the sensi in your system. The sun will rise soon, so the music changes to reggae for the wind down. But all you partygoers protest, making the selector rewind and come again with "So leave me alone! I ain't going home! Let me party!" (Rose 2016). You laugh and sing along. This is joy. This is healing. This is release.

As people from historically and currently oppressed backgrounds navigating tough realities, we often don't get to experience sustained moments of happiness or restoration, like the aforementioned scene, unless we create it for ourselves. At the hands of (neo)colonialism, sexism, anti-Blackness, capitalism, anti-queerness, and overall kyriarchy, our bodies have often been painted by violent histories and present-day realities as sites of excavation, terror, and labor, instead of homes of desire, pleasure, and enjoyment. In efforts to bring about social change, many people highlight how Black, Brown, and Indigenous peoples—and persons of marginalized a/genders and a/sexualities in particular—are treated as disposable and sacrificial (Tuck 2009, 414). Of course, emphasizing this has brought much-needed attention, acknowledgment, and benefits. However, it has also produced harm through the ramifications of labeling communities as "disadvantaged," "vulnerable," and "underrepresented," instead of being explicit in addressing systems as exploitative, negligent, or violent. Such damage-centered narratives cannot be the only stories about our communities or the primary ways to enable change (Tuck 2009). The pleasure, healing, and liberation that we continue to claim for ourselves (even via the physical and mental health benefits of temporary things like a weekend fete) must be included in the stories we tell and the change we facilitate. Honoring multidimensionality in our existence and expression is key to catalyzing and reclaiming individual and collective healing and advancement.

The proliferation of harmful narratives about Black, Brown, and Indigenous communities has continued in the COVID-19 pandemic. Beginning in March 2020, many of us went inside and stayed home, sometimes alone, unable to spend time with loved ones, unable to lime with our friends, unable to watch the pandemic response without anxiety or fear. Most macabre was seeing united states–based[3] media and research further one-dimensional stories by focusing on Black people moving through and dying in an intricate web of biological, social, and physical violence and being "overrepresented" among coronavirus mortality rates (Cowger et al. 2020). For sure, this discourse is not unique to the united states—the precarity of life as a Black person has been a long-standing global reality since the earliest days of european colonizers enslaving Africans. But Black folks and our coconspirators reject this as an unchangeable truism. Recent examples of contesting the pervasiveness of such perilous existence include homegrown protests against police brutality throughout Africa and the Black Diaspora,[4] such as in Trinidad,[5] Brazil,[6] and Nigeria.[7] Through spotlighting atrocities and calling for rest, reparations, and abolition within local systems and in transnational solidarity efforts, Black peoples and their accomplices follow a rich historical practice of self-reclamation, resistance against oppression, and actualization of liberation. Conceding the ubiquity of Black death as a central issue transcending geopolitical borders and simultaneously rejecting it as status quo, we ask ourselves, "As members of the Black Caribbean Diaspora, how might we understand our identities and capacities to enrich pleasure and healing for ourselves and each other during and beyond the COVID-19 pandemic?"

Beginning to answer this requires us to translate cultural knowledge across boundaries and generations to engage in passed-down and remixed practices to restore ourselves in our current locations. Equipped with the teachings of our displaced predecessors, who strategized to ensure survival and repossess freedom in lands that were not their ancestral homes (Sutherland et al. 2013), we build upon practices that provide emotional, spiritual, and bodily sustenance. These help us deal with the everyday realities of life under oppressive systems (like the educational institution conferring our doctoral degrees) and hold on to the assurances of community and self-care that enable us to move beyond surviving to get to flourishing (Powerful, Jolly, and Stephens 2020). We know that we can't do pleasure and healing work alone. Just like successful events need a team of organizers, selectors, cooks, feters, decorators, etc. to guarantee maximum vibes and freeupness,[8] we need to rely on each other.

During this critical pandemic juncture, it's important for us to think about Caribbean culture, scholarship, and practices with intentions other than the valid reason that they are core to our identities and academic work. The Caribbean's geopolitical history of being exploited by multinational corporations and (neo)colonizing countries (which use it as a factory, playground, and slaughterhouse) has facilitated the (1) creation of a Diaspora that is almost as populous as the Caribbean itself (IOM 2021) and (2) inequitable/unsustainable development of a region whose global contributions are often dismissed because it is seen as a "small player"[9] on the world stage. With COVID-19 in the united states being purposely mismanaged (Diamond 2020),[10] usonians[11] are flocking to the Caribbean to escape (Burleigh 2020), callously spreading coronavirus to places with limited pandemic management capacity—in large part due to u.s. interference[12]—and eerily replicating the colonial spread of disease from colonizers to Indigenous and enslaved African communities. There is a violent, inescapable interconnectedness between the Caribbean and the united states that signifies for us how we cannot hold only our Caribbeanness or our "americanization" as we process how we're living through this year. And this interconnectedness reveals why we consider it necessary to share our experiences of taking care of our Black Caribbean Diasporic selves during the pandemic, existing "in that in-between space that is neither here nor there" (Boyce-Davies 1994, 1).

Grounding Through Ancestral Guides and Patnas

These musings are further grounded in the fact that we come from a heritage of Black Caribbean people who have long engaged in cultivating individual and collective restoration that centers embodied desires and capacities for healing and pleasure. By design, we bring Black Caribbean women (familiar in familial, spiritual, and academic ways) into this conversation about how holding on to (even the smallest moments of) joy and healing is relevant to the current time. An example is this essay's title; it is a remix of Calypso Rose's 2016 song "Leave Me Alone," whose lyrics also bring an end to our essay's opening scene. This Trinidadian artist is renowned not only for her musical dexterity and longevity but also because she is unapologetic about her autonomy, vocal about her sensuality, and adamant about her enjoyment of life. Just as we are led by the voice of this calypsonian on the dance floor and in our lives, we rely on ancestral guides to move us through spaces of pleasure and restoration. Adding our voices as we build upon the legacies of Black women's explorations of self and community care, we seek to enrich our own joy and healing through slowness, dancing, and cooking during the coronavirus pandemic. This matters because trying to follow pandemic etiquette makes it easier to disconnect/dissociate and harder to cope, when what would serve us better would be to be present with ourselves and process the uncertainty of everything. Reengaging with intimacy and connection as a necessary part of healing during COVID-19 counters the idea that we have to isolate in order to stay healthy.

One of our primary guides is Black Grenadian/Bajan lesbian imaginator and disruptor Audre Lorde. Like us, she traverses different fluid identities, including that of a Caribbean Diasporic woman who sees the region as both a physical and spiritual home. In much of her work, Lorde highlights the complex identities of Diasporic peoples of African descent and a yearning for community and longing for home. The cadence of her fluidity also illuminates for us her perspectives on negotiating belonging, understanding pleasure, and (re)claiming power. This is palpable in *Zami: A New Spelling of My Name*, a biomythography in which she shares how the intimate relationships with the women in her life, including her Grenadian mother, shape her understanding of love and thrival (Lorde 1982). In addition, one of Lorde's most cited works, *Uses of the Erotic: The Erotic as Power*, affirms for us that being in touch with the erotic, a source of knowledge and power that lies between self-understanding and the turmoil of our most intense feelings (1978), can only be achieved through connections across interwoven political, spiritual, and sensual desires (Gill 2018, 9). So we reflect and apply.

Together we draw on many scholars, who also build on Lorde's work, to frame and contextualize our experiences during COVID-19. We see these folks as our winin' and bruk out patnas who move in sync with us under the influence of the harmonies and resonance central to Lorde's germinal theorizing. Their scholarship gifts us the language to understand, contextualize, and describe our experiences and permit us to consider what pleasure in the face of multifaceted oppressions looks like for folks like us. For example, we see our writing as (1) tending to Dr. Omise'eke Natasha Tinsley's call to challenge traditional archives and develop Black feminist epistemologies that uncover our histories (Allen and Tinsley 2012, 249) and (2) invoking M. Jacqui Alexander's notion of "sacred memory" (2005). As such, we build on the intimacies of the Black Caribbean relations to self and others that Lorde highlights, by spending time with our current experiences and relating them to concepts, such as the erotic and fluid Diasporic identities, that we have found useful in helping us to be reflexive.

Together with our patnas and guides we center ourselves in a cultural legacy of Black women who ensured survival by asserting agency and envisioning freedom. Following the example of the playful engagement between Lorde and Pat Parker (Lorde and Parker 2018), over a few weeks we emailed each other letters that navigate home, identity, belonging, care, slowness, food, family, healing, and dance in meaningful ways that our usual interactions via video chat, messaging apps, social media, and other instantaneous, urgency-inducing platforms don't facilitate. The letters allowed us to (1) craft with care words that fit what we wish to share, (2) revel in each other's thoughts, and (3) take time between responses. They are also glimpses into our embodied archives,[13] which are connected to our moving through time and space.

We combine the intimacy of letter writing with analytic reflections, to explore how we restore our bodies and how our bodies restore us, physically, spiritually, and mentally. In this way, we witness and share our embodiment of our desires for more pleasurable and liberated existences. These epistles document strategy and tactic; they are documented application and reclamation of Black Caribbean people's agency in sustaining our ability to survive and flourish in the face of oppression and existential threats. And this is important because the lessons we are learning at this moment force reflection we have not engaged in prior, even though we live in such close proximity to disease, violence, and colonialism (Endia Hayes, in conversation with authors, November 5, 2020). We hope that our readers will be inspired by our use of letter writing, the intimate relation building, and how we connect that to healing (through our expansion of the view that healing is traditionally associated with biological well-being) to transform thoughts of what joy and restoration can look like during COVID-19. Our contribution showcases a practical way of having this multifaceted approach toward pandemic coping practices, which will be pivotal as we move toward imaging future modes of healing for the generations of Black Caribbean Diasporic folks to come.[14]

Embodied Epistles and Sacred Memories

Epistle Pairing I
September 2, 2020
Dear Sherine,
I had my dissertation committee meeting this morning, and though it went fine, my energy felt so depleted afterward. I tried to get some work done right after, and within an hour my eyes began to gloss over. Naturally, I turned on some Dexta Daps and spent a few hours danc-

ing. My roommate hasn't been around since March; I'm guessing he went home because of COVID. What this means for me, however, is that my kitchen floor is my own personal dance studio. Whew girl, the way I was flippin' and rollin' and splittin' and kickin', you'd think something was wrong with me. I definitely chuckled at myself a few times, because I promise you, I looked ridiculous. But here's the thing—it made me realize how much I miss silliness and playfulness and just simply doing things for my own entertainment. The "quick break" turned into the entire day off. I put in my headphones and the day just escaped me. I practiced my routine for the workshop me and Gia are teaching later this month (it's a collaboration with another brand, and I am super excited!). I listened to Masego and just got lost in my thoughts . . . I feel like I haven't allowed myself to have this type of release in so long. I think I assumed that structuring one-hour breaks throughout the day would be enough, but it's clearly not. . . . So my spiritual cup feels so much fuller today. As I'm eating my corn soup and writing this, I'm realizing how many more of these days I want and need. I'm at the point where I'm thinking a lot about the future as I apply to postdoctoral programs. And while I'm not sure where to find a career that centers dance and mental health / dancehall instruction / flexibility to attend Carnivals—essentially all parts of me, I am certain that I want a future with more days like today.

Love, O

September 7, 2020
Hey Onisha!
Congrats on getting through your dissertation committee meeting! It sounds like you might have been pushing yourself more than your mind wanted you to, so I'm glad you trusted your intuition and switched to engaging your body in movement. And raaeeeee to having the apartment to yourself! Now you know there is nothing wrong with puttin' yuh back in it and bussin' a split! You had fun! That's all

that matters . . . I feel you so much on missing silliness and playfulness for yourself. It's so easy to neglect that when it feels like the world's going to shit, and it's important to hold tight to it once we can reclaim that. Shoutout to you for taking the day "off" to dance and flow. Music is so powerful for our bodies. And I've seen Masego's name but haven't listened to their music. Let me pause and put on a song . . . Okay, I'm back. Masego is a vibe! And they have Jamaican heritage! Okay, this is today's mood; I'll channel you so I can have a contemplative, creative, "pleasure is greater than productivity" day! Also, you thinking one-hour breaks would be enough definitely resonates. It really isn't enough. I read an article on surge capacity depletion and how our bodies weren't meant to process this much stress. It made me reflect on the rollercoaster of emotions/symptoms I've had since lockdown, and how, even with all the breaks I take, I have been feeling completely exhausted. So since I've been in Jamaica, taking physical and emotional space to both process and disconnect from the trauma of being Black in the u.s., I've been channeling the Nap Ministry's[15] call to center rest. I've found joy again in taking naps, in lying down and letting my mind wander . . . stillness feels so good! So YES to your spiritual cup feeling fuller. You deserve fullness, replenishment, AND rest! You deserve more of those kinds of days, AND a career that centers all parts of you. But . . . you may have to create it. It's scary, but you know what? We gotta invest in our own Black futures, boo! There's so much world building, futures building, to be done. Let's get it.

Nuff Love, Sherine

Sacred Memories I: Movement

If you've ever experienced a Caribbean family gathering, then you know the scene of multiple generations huddled in one house with some cookin', some limin', and some winin'. Being in such intimate proximity to family members curating pleasure and joy together, which often changed depending on whose auntie was hosting that week, we learned what "home" can look and feel like. Seeing our grandmothers put the pot spoon down when their favorite song came on to "catch a wine" in between cooking for everyone also demonstrated the release that a quick dance could give. Onisha draws on these familiar experiences in her letter as she holds space for the depletion and fulfillment she experiences through working, PhD-ing, dancing, and resting.

Through employing Tuck's conceptualization of desire being "about longing, about a present that is enriched by both the past and the future" and as "integral to our humanness" (2009, 417), we can see that rather than sitting with exhaustion, Onisha asserts agency in moving toward the fullness she hungers for that fosters her own healing and wellness. She feels the toll of working during a taxing time and pressures of "being productive" and pauses to draw on her body and art to fill her "spiritual cup." Much like the grandmother putting the pot spoon down to catch a wine, through turning toward play and pleasure, movement and stillness, Onisha produces a sacred space for herself where she can feel a sense of release and dream of a future that holds all parts of her humanity.

Drawing on the body and dance for restoration and release is a familiar practice to Black Caribbean people. Jamaican dancehall, for instance, accepts the coexistence of the sacred and profane in what often serves as an embodied spiritual place where "something overtakes you," similar to "catching the spirit" in some Christian traditions (Brown 2017). Onisha's description of her dancing and her comment that "you'd think something was wrong with me" speaks to a sense of release so powerful that it teeters the boundaries of the spiritual in relation to the transformation she feels. This day of intimate time with her body and creating a sacred space in opposition to the capitalist ideologies of productivity is an intertwining of the political-sensual-spiritual (Gill 2018, 10) that leads to self-understanding and a standard for pleasure that she aims for in the future (Lorde 1978).

While Onisha's movement via dancing occurs in one space, Sherine's movement is via traveling between two countries. What is not shared in the letter, but was shared between us in conversation, is that this homecoming was an intentional self-repatriation, for health and well-being, family reconnection, and spiritual survival, planned years in advance of the pandemic. Sherine admits that she is giving herself space away from her Diasporic location to restore and get back to herself, both invoking and deconstructing what Angelique Nixon calls a transnational Diasporic homespace (2015, 65),[16] in a metaphorical dance between lands. This contributes to Sherine both being at home inside her body and her body now existing in home, representing Nixon's concept of "Black female travel," which reflects how Caribbean people navigate harmful systems like neo-colonialism, and asserting "radical Black subjectivity and feminist postcolonial resistance" (2015, 28). This movement across geographies presents a common grappling with identity and authenticity, (neo)colonialism and imperialism, and migration and mobility that resonates with our own tensions of being both from and away from the Caribbean (Nixon 2015). Sherine's homecoming is an endeavor to (re)define connection with a land she frequently returns to and leaves often; a space of release with newfound joys and desires; and a political act of self-preservation and sensual gratification through naps, stillness, and music.

Both Sherine and Onisha validate that the Caribbean is no "small space," as it is often portrayed, but that Caribbean spaces are extensive, lovingly created and re-created, and not limited by geography (Boyce-Davies 2013, 1–2). Our experiences mirror the long trajectory of Caribbean peoples moving, curating, and defining space for themselves across the Diaspora. During a time defined by restriction of physical movement, we create expansiveness for replenishment and manifest intimacy beyond physical touch. Safety and health during a crisis through our Black Caribbean Diasporic lens do not need to be devoid of movement or intimacy but, rather, they are integrated into imaginaries of healing that center our well-being.

Epistle Pairing II
September 8, 2020
Mawnin O!
Girl. I feel so at peace right now. More at home, inside and outside my body, than I have in a long time. I'm in the middle of quarantine. My family checks in all the time, asking if they can drop off food, or if I'm bored. And I have to laugh and tell them that I am good. That I am better than I have been in a long time. That just being in JA already has my hair shining, skin clearing, and inflammation diminishing. . . . This morning I didn't fight the early sunrise. I got out of bed, steeped fever grass for tea, and put on music, reflecting on how grateful I am for this homecoming. Corona cases are skyrocketing here too. I feel I jumped out of the fire (of the u.s.) and into the frying pan. But . . . nowhere is perfect. And nowhere will be free from the influence of u.s. empire. And I am still a student, embedded in one of the most capitalist, imperialist institutions in the world. So . . . I'll be in my frying pan, dancing (cue Chi Ching Ching, "roast fry, fry, roast fry fry"), making the best of my situation, loving up my family, working on my thesis, and deliberately choosing joy. . . . Anyway, after teatime, I turned up the music as my soundtrack to cooking. A little Chloe x Halle "Do It (Remix)" as I wined while cutting up garlic, tomato, onions, sweet pepper, and scotch bonnet and marveled at the wet, fragrant chunkiness with my fingers. Some Spice "Inches" as I swung my dreads along my back before sautéing the aromatics. A little Jada Kingdom "Budum" as I mixed in shredded saltfish. And a tups of Shenseea "Sure Sure" as I added chopped callaloo, covering to steam until done. I danced for an hour, stealing bites of breakfast between verses. It felt so good to move and embrace comfort in my surroundings, to know that in the middle of a pandemic, this perpetual nomad could finally

feel at home. Before today, I'd only been able to buss out short dancing stints before feeling unmotivated and dejected. But today was a
breakthrough. Today was a day when warmth became a way of being
and not just a feeling. When my body released the tension of the sci-fi
nightmare-come-true playing out around us by absorbing the sounds
of Black/Caribbean women enjoying their bodies and pleasure and
just vibing and rocking and swaying. I think I'm getting back to me,
O. Lemme dance some more to that!

                                                          Nuff Love, Sherine

September 14, 2020
Hi, Hello, Good Morning!
Wowww! Your letter made me smile ear to ear. It's so beautiful to hear
you describe what being at home feels like. Not just physically at home,
but also spiritually, mentally, emotionally—all of it. I am so excited
for you. And yessss to your body recognizing its home and showing
up and out! And hey, the frying pan ain't ever do me dirty, only good
things come out of that—saltfish, fry bake, plantains—whew! I'll take
frying pan over fire any day. . . . Your description of the gentleness you
allowed in your day is everything we need to be reminded of, particularly in contexts where we're still faced with demands for "productivity" at work or school. Moments to dance, sip slowly on tea, move
to the sizzle of the meal we're cooking—everything that allows us to
slow down and truly experience life fully is so necessary. I always say,
"Our bodies know us best." When you're tired, your body will let you
know. When you need movement or ease, your body will give you
all the cues you need. . . . The other day I saw this question posed by
Tricia Hersey: "How can we access pleasure & joy & liberation, if we're
too tired to experience it?"[17] The gentleness that you bring into your
day is precisely what refuels and rejuvenates you, and I hope that you
continue to have opportunities to bring more of that into your space,
and, by extension, experience all of the pleasure, joy, and liberation

that comes with it. I am proud of you for deliberately choosing joy. I hope that you have more days to choose joy, and more places, people, and systems that center and celebrate you doing so. You are getting back to yourself, and I'm so here for this rejuvenating journey!

Love you! O

Sacred Memories II: Creating Home

One of the defining contours of Caribbean Diasporic communities is food, connecting people from Jamaica to Panama to Canada, and beyond. Where there is access to Caribbean cuisine (di real food), there is cultural community and home. Now situated in her birthplace, Sherine's process of making callaloo and saltfish, a beloved family dish, using local ingredients (in particular, the fresh vegetable seasoning base common to most Caribbean dishes), brings the physical concept of home together with a desire to embrace and apply passed-down cooking methods and savor robust, familiar flavors. Being able to prepare a cultural meal with all the ingredients in the comfort of a kitchen with space to dance is a restorative part of Sherine's journey of (re)creating home and returning home to herself. Her naming of each ingredient, "marvel[ing] in the wet, fragrant chunkiness with [her] fingers," and stealing bites in between song verses reflects Sumita Dutta's description of cooking as an act of "evoking recipes, flavors, seasonal, and geographic foods" that also conjures "desire through specificity, ancestral knowledge (such-and-such's recipe), and orients us to our life force, through taste" (2016, 6).

Sitting with Sherine's intimate connection to the food she is making and feeling and smelling, which allows her to spend time in the erotic plane and delve into her pleasures, reminds us of Tao Leigh Goffe's description of food as "an archive of global desires" (2019, 31). Goffe interpolates depictions of colonizers "traveling" out of wants for exploration (really, conquest) with the freedom/unfreedom to eat whatever/whenever one wants for enslaved Africans and indentured

South Asians on Caribbean plantations, thus alluding to and affirming a complex relationship between desire and food for Black and Brown peoples (2019). We also see this notion of desire and food in Dutta's understanding of cooking's healing power and its role as mind, body, and spirit work (2016), which furthers this notion of the longing and belonging infused into Sherine's meal preparation. Cooking as a practice and experience among Caribbean people is a sensuous and sensual experience, and this is clear in the environment Sherine has created for herself where she feels peace and comfort and warmth as a way of being. She is deliberate in seeking joy and pleasure in family and cooking, drawing on familial and navigational capital (Yosso 2005) to cope with her current reality. This very engagement with the sensual and spiritual is an act of political resistance to access pleasure and healing, however fleeting or temporary they may be.

In her response, Onisha talks about how the frying pan has always done right by her in its use of preparing Caribbean culinary delights. This reframing of Sherine's "out of the fire . . . and into the frying pan" metaphor highlights the fact that while coronavirus cases are increasing in her new location, she can still coat herself in a little goodness (and with good food). This playful insistence underscores the shared Diasporic cultural connections between us, and how we maneuver positions that often seem at odds with one another in order to claim pleasure and healing for ourselves. To further understand this, we uplift adrienne maree brown's explanation of pleasure as all of the experiences in life that make us feel alive, bring us happiness, and allow us to access transcendence, which deliberately extends Lorde's relating of the erotic to pleasure and feeling alive and sex (brown 2019, 22). Our Diasporic identities and capacities to create home within and outside of ourselves are connected to our desires to be happier, healthier, and freer by engaging in healing in whatever ways we can, including food and dance as we see in our letters. Creating and coming home for Sherine means more frequent breakthroughs, more time spent dancing and moving, and more time processing and transcending limitations to the many possible manifestations of pleasure.

Epistle Pairing III
September 17, 2020
Hey Sherine,

This has been . . . a week. One positive thing is that I had my first (virtual) session for the Dancehall Queens course I'm teaching at Tufts! The students were so incredibly thoughtful and engaged, and it has me geeked for the semester. I see them already wrestling with how dancehall can simultaneously be a space for women to reclaim sexual authority and still have much work needed for everyone to be safe and included. I think one of the best parts is that a lot of them have never had exposure to Dancehall, so for their introduction to be through this liberatory and Caribbean feminist lens is just so rare and exciting. As thrilled as I am about the course, I definitely am feeling at capacity and on the peak of burnout. Things feel like they're going at 100 MPH, and I haven't had time to slow down. This has me in a mini-existential-crisis mode of wondering if academia is for me, given how blurry boundaries are between work and personal life. The biggest way I've been able to slow time is cooking, though, since I gotta eat! So, I've been trying to make my meal time sacred. I'll put headphones on, play some gospel or lovers rock (there's no in between!) and take my time. I think cooking is the only time I'm not staring at a screen. It feels so good. . . . This week I made chicken curry, and I surprised myself with how easy it was (this is a dish I've only cooked three times before). I mixed the masala, curry powder, and geera like it was second nature, and I didn't have to meticulously measure por-. tions. I doubt I was even thinking much because I was so focused on Beres Hammond singing "remember those days they used to make you rockaway" and swaying in the kitchen (but not enough to get caught dancing if my roommate walked in). I think about how I'd be in awe whenever I saw my grandma cooking this so effortlessly. That woman could be cooking a full three-course meal, catching up on soap operas, and talking on the phone all at once. Now I'm like, "I'm well on my way to being at that level." I definitely need many more years of practice, but I felt so much closer to home making that dish, especially given that I've been on lockdown away from my family. I hope your week's been okay. Let me know what you been cheffin' up!

Love, O

September 30, 2020

Onishaaaaa!

I feel you on this being a WEEK! Congratulations on completing your first class! You are well on your way to blooming further into your Dr. Rude Gyal essence. And yes, yes, yes to engaging and thoughtful students. I can only imagine the mixed emotions as you anticipated how your students would respond to you as a first-time lecturer. I'm sending you all the positive vibes for a beautiful, mutually beneficial learning experience. . . . And I say it at least every other day, but this pandemic definitely has us in a reverse time warp / twilight zone. So I echo your sentiments on things moving rapidly. If you can, try to make space for yourself to deeply experience the existential crisis as a valid phase of your adulthood journey, while being more direct with yourself and others about your boundaries . . . and mmhmm! Cooking is a time-tested way of slowing down so that we can experience the making and savoring of food with as many senses as possible. You gotta eat and nourish and heal your body! We may have to fight over "chicken curry" vs. "curry chicken," the same way we fight over "whine" vs. "wine," but big ups to you in getting closer to that aspirational level of effortlessly finessing meals! That same awe your grandma inspired in you, I'm sure, will be the same awe you inspire in yourself and in others once they experience your slow-crafted and intentionally curated culinary skills. What things were coming up for you as you felt yourself getting closer to your grandma's level? What feelings did your food invoke in you as you cooked and savored it? What were your ancestors whispering in your ears as you added each new ingredient? You may have been on lockdown away from your family, but I'm sure the spirits were guiding you. Axé, friend.

Nuff Love, Sherine

Sacred Memories III: Time-Warping

Caribbean people have superpowers when it comes to warping time. We often operate in CPT—Caribbean People Time; the radical act of having time be whatever di rass you want it to be and not letting anyone else dictate it for you. So the party starts at eight o'clock? That means we showin' up at midnight. This relationship to the amorphousness of time has been a prominent feature for us in 2020, evidenced by Sherine's references to "reverse time warp" and "twilight zone" and Onisha's description of a particular instance during the pandemic as "going at 100 MPH." These characterizations of time indicate that it is not making sense in the usual ways. So, through her letter, we see how Onisha absorbs this warp as she slows down to resist capitalist values of productivity and create intentional time for herself.

Onisha shares how she craves slowness, to ensure she does not reach a state of burnout, which she is only able to find through cooking. This time spent crafting and savoring with all her senses, while making a meal that connects her to family and heritage, is a deliberate form of physical and spiritual deceleration. In the famous words of Auntie Maxine Waters, Onisha is "reclaiming her time" (*Washington Post* 2017). And Sherine's assertion that the ancestors/spirits are whispering in Onisha's ears and guiding her, in response to the desire to get on her grandmother's level of replenishment and multitasking during sacred meal time, is a loving acknowledgment of this time-bending experience of cooking as an emotional and impactful process (again, evoking Dutta's cooking and healing pedagogy). Even Onisha's music choices of gospel and lovers rock demonstrate the spiritual and the sensual meeting and existing at the same time. So we read Onisha's letter as documentation of creating a deliberate, fulfilling, healing space for herself, and Sherine's response as bearing witness to this intentional act. This act is tied to the political; it's an active carving of space in systems that cause harm and do not allow wellness.

In this time-warped, twilight-zone here and now, such an act controls our environment, with guidance from our ancestors and community, to create a new present. Carole Boyce-Davies's definition of twilight zones as "spaces of transformation from one condition to another, one location to another, and the sometimes newly created emotional, physical, and conceptual space that then becomes another identified location" and "scary spaces of loss but also of gain" (2013, 11–12) is an apt conceptualization for this COVID-19 era. Boyce-Davies's assertion that these twilight zones and liminal, yet expansive, locations constitute a Caribbean space speaks to both Sherine's feelings on how different time has become and Onisha's leaning into Caribbean People Time. Onisha's transformation of time through slowness and ancestral/familial connection offers a new "location" of being, or reality, in which she can revel.

This very analysis of our letters requires an intentional engagement with and return to the "twilight zone." Here we reflect on where our minds and bodies directed us earlier this year. We spend precious moments with these memories and let them guide us now, months after they happened, as reminders of our identities and capacities. And we take time to consider other patnas and guides whose presence and influence encourage us, as we notice how they've also experienced similar realities and emotions. Our twilight zone is unlimited by any particular moment, capacious enough for loss and gain, and replete with new ways of being as we navigate the physical locations we are restricted to during COVID-19.

Moving Beyond This Moment

As Black Caribbean Diasporic people who navigate multiple spaces at the same time, we both feel a pull toward home: Sherine physically returns to reconnect and rejuvenate, while Onisha spiritually immerses herself through memory and culture. Regardless of location, our identities ground us and enable us to affirm each other in shared practices of restoration. We witness each other learning to speed up or slow down time, engage in physical and figurative movement for rejuvenation, and tap into our intimate relationships with home in ways that serve our needs for more fulfilling ways of being. And we understand our capacities to enrich pleasure and healing as regenerative and grounded in physical and emotional nourishment. So we see all that we draw upon to both restore ourselves and understand our processes as relevant to coping during COVID-19, as these processes assert that we already have the tools within us to secure our existence both now and in the future beyond the pandemic.

Dutta tells us that "capitalistic models of wellness rob us of a healing that is wide, generative, and tied to the whole truth of the land that holds our bodies" (2016, 3). COVID-19 responses have been so detrimental largely because they privilege a capitalist system that does not care about the survival of Black, Brown, and Indigenous communities. Since March 2020, we have received mixed messages from government and health officials about how to stay healthy and safe during the pandemic. Many of these messages reflect elements of white supremacist culture,[18] capitalist values, or the euro-american biomedical model,[19] which cannot be applied to all sociocultural contexts. For example, communications around isolating/quarantining and postponing/sacrificing joy (1) relate to individualism, which is counter to many community-oriented cultures; (2) deny people outlets for mourning and celebration, which are key to mental health and well-being; and (3) do not encourage alternate ways of reducing

COVID-19 transmission if they're not deemed (euro-american approved) "best practices" (Macoloo 2020). Another example is the advice to use this "extra" time "wisely," now that many people are spending more time indoors, which prioritizes productivity and urgency to get more things done, when what we need to be doing is resting to recover from myriad traumas. As public health practitioners studying at an institution in the united states, we have been taught the rationale behind this. We know that these advisories do not always serve Black, Brown, and Indigenous communities who have their own means of attending to physical, mental, spiritual, and emotional health during crises. Folks who have been harmed by systems of oppression all have tools and resources to draw on for thinking about healing, tools that are tied to our connection between our bodies and the lands we inhabit, to return to Dutta's framing.

This restorative writing has enabled us to move closer to the individuals we desire to be: creative, caring, thoughtful, expressive, dancing beings who revel in food, sensuality, and family. Doing this together has fostered healing in our friendship, while aiding in our own unlearning of internalized damage-centered foci of self and community. Through this, we have been making space for versions of ourselves we feel we lost while navigating young adulthood, connecting with playfulness and healing via our imaginations and creativity, and reading about ancestral practices to reflect on how we embody such legacies. Holding sacred memories in our embodied archives created by/for ourselves as Black Caribbean people allows for the reclamation, healing, and support that governmental negligence in managing the COVID-19 pandemic has constricted.

Giving ourselves room to legitimize our processing and recollection of how we restore ourselves and how our bodies restore us—as we are made to slow down, observe, and feel—and use this as documentation and a site of healing, disrupts the euro-american academic notions of "objectivity" and "distance." Tinsley frames the paucity of historical documentation and the need for creative responses as a legitimate way to represent Black women's histories, citing, for example, Saidiya Hartman's use of creative narratives to fill gaps in the archives through her concept of "critical fabulation" (Allen and Tinsley 2012).[20] Educational scholarship from the euro-american traditions in which we are embedded could never suffice for a comprehensive recording of our healing and restoration. So we extend on Hartman and Tinsley by creating our own archives of our experiences, interwoven with creative narratives.

We see intimacy, introspection, and community as central sites of knowing. Allen and Tinsley (2012) build on this idea of intimate knowledge by invoking Alexander's contention that "water overflows with memory . . . emotional memory, bodily memory, sacred memory" (2005, 290). This is one way to express the need to develop a Black feminist epistemology to uncover submerged histories that euro-american historiographies cannot, and will not, validate. Further, this development and acknowledgment of embodied archives is a way for us to employ our own desire-based approaches for how we and other Black Caribbean folks can move through the pandemic in ways that center our bodies and cultural relations.

COVID-19 presented us with unprecedented daily realities. Yet we find that all around us, mainstream channels continue to propagate trite, one-dimensional narratives of Black people. Alternatives that (re)center Black pleasures and the hope to exist beyond coronavirus *and* despite systems of oppression will carry us through times of crisis. We suspect that we would not be making these considerations in such acute ways if we were not in the middle of a pandemic. Coronavirus is making everything feel more pressing and heightened as it has caused a halt to the world as we know/knew it. So becoming more thoughtful about slowing down and caring for our bodies is a valid response, not just related to this pandemic, but to any time. We contend that this process of conversation, reflection, and analysis is useful for pandemics and beyond.

"Cyah Leave We Alone, We Rel Stayin' Home"

We wind down this essay with Calypso Rose blaring from the speakers, sipping spirited drinks, and winin' slow as she prolongs each word: "We havin a ball! Nobody can't stop we! No not at all!" By remixing Calypso Rose's 2016 song "Leave Me Alone" for this essay's title, we cheekily uplift the fact that even though COVID-19 has us staying at home, separate from one another, we can't leave each other alone. We are in this— everything that "this" signifies—together. Mothers and grandmothers, calypso queens, and scholar-artist-activists have all been a source of learning for us in cultivating our own pleasure and healing. As Black Caribbean Diasporic beings, we have so many folks winin' beside us and intentionally choosing joy and restoration. A cherished example is that of Caribbean people who participate(d) in Carnival celebrations/ rituals to work through and heal from their pain and trauma (Henry 2019), remix(ed) and slow(ed) time to revel in the present moment, and curate(d) spaces for themselves that know no geographic boundaries.

Caribbean Diasporic communities have long engaged with trauma and harms of multiple systems in between worlds and locations, and they illustrate what it means to find healing through engaging with pleasure. We cherish and uplift Alisha B. Wormsley's declaration that "there are Black People in the Future" (n.d.). Neither enslavement, nor brutality, nor pandemics will wipe us / wear us / weed us out. And COVID-19 is neither a motivator for nor an end point in this avowal. It is a catalyst, added to the middle of this maelstrom created by destructive people and oppressive systems, that has produced this critical moment necessitating (re)new(ed) actions. We may have to be inside, for a (much) long(er) time, but we will continue to act, to resist, to heal, to restore.

Notes

1. Jamaican term for the person who selects the music (specifically riddims) to play (similar to a DJ in other cultures).

2. Jamaican dancehall music from the early 2000s. Dancehall is a genre of music originating in Jamaica and is influenced by a mix of many genres, including reggae.

3. This decapitalization follows Audre Lorde's tradition of using lowercase letters for *united states* and *america*.

4. Throughout the essay, the capitalization of *Diaspora* indicates it grammatically as a proper noun and politically as a separate, yet connected, identity category and social grouping with a specific history and traits that don't render it as a sidekick to the "original" social group.

5. On June 8, 2020, in solidarity with protests against police murders of u.s. Black people, organizers in Trinidad gathered to decry state violence against Black Trinis. On June 27, the Trinidad and Tobago Police Service shot and killed Noel Diamond, Joel Jacob, and Israel Moses Clinton in the Morvant neighborhood of Port of Spain. On June 30, Ornella Greaves was shot and murdered at a subsequent protest against police violence. These killings in turn sparked more protests and critiques of the police (Christopher 2020; Steuart 2020; Loop News 2020).

6. In June 2020, the murder of João Pedro Mattos Pinto in Brazil, a week before the murder of George Floyd in the united states, reinvigorated the #VidasNegrasImportam demonstrations against police violence and demands for justice that initially amplified after police killed a Black Brazilian at the supermarket in February 2019. Additional protests took place in November 2020 after white security guards killed a Black man (Liscia 2020; Davinchi 2020).

7. In early October 2020, after the circulation of videos of officers from the Special Anti-Robbery Squad (SARS) murdering, exploiting, and kidnapping people, Nigerians organized demonstrations to #EndSARS. On October 20, officers attempted to suppress dissent by turning off lights, removing cameras, and shooting protestors in what is now known as the Lekki Tollgate Massacre (Osakwe 2020).

8. We define *freeupness* as the active quality of embodying freeness through outward expression of joy.

9. And by small player, we mean that the Caribbean is treated as a political pawn.

10. Using a flawed interpretation of the public health concept of herd immunity to achieve the ulterior motive of furthering capitalistic ideals, government officials endangered the health and well-being of people living in the united states, especially those from historically and currently oppressed communities.

11. This is a more accurate synonym for *americans*, given that the term is most used to represent people living in the united states and not those living in other parts of the Western Hemisphere.

12. For example, in April 2020, the united states blocked the Cayman Islands, Barbados, and the Bahamas from receiving medical devices, personal protective equipment, and ventilators to help with the COVID-19 response (Charles and Harris 2020). Another example of u.s. interference took place in October 2020, when the ambassador to Jamaica threatened the island's government with financial consequences and denial of aid for extreme weather events recovery if Jamaica continued with plans to acquire 5G technology from China (Pate 2020).

13. In "Jah Kingdom: Rastafarians, Tanzania, and Pan-Africanism in the Age of Decolonization," Monique Bedasse uses "embodied archive" to describe how Rastafarians hold knowledge within themselves that they travel with, knowledge that is not always shared with researchers or written down for physical documentation (cited in Moore 2018).

14. For examples of contemporary means of contributing to intracommunity archival and actualization work that centers healing and pleasure, check out (1) the Caribbean Women Healers Project, led by Dr. Ana-Maurine Lara and Dr. Alaí Reyes-Santos at the University of Oregon, a digital humanities collaboration that engages in critical research through deep listening and oral histories; and (2) the Carib Healing Collective, led by Ruth Jeannoel, Samantha Daley, and Bianca Campbell, who provide workshops and education on Caribbean herbalism.

15. Founded by Tricia Hersey in 2016, the Nap Ministry is an organization that uplifts the healing power of naps through installations, workshops, and community organizing.

16. In other words, locating one's self simultaneously in multiple spaces, which for Sherine is both a Caribbean and an americanized Black space.

17. Nap Ministry 2020.

18. For a full list of the characteristics of white supremacy culture, see Jones and Okun 2001.

19. The biomedical model of medicine and healing that has become a global standard due to european imperialism treats the mind and body as separate and distinct, but does not incorporate the spirit or spirituality, and by extension does not incorporate sensuality or the erotic, which are paramount to the traditional health and well-being models of Black, Brown, and Indigenous communities. This renders the biomedical model limited and, often times, culturally irrelevant (Sutherland et al. 2013).

20. In "Venus in Two Acts," Hartman (2008) uses critical fabulation as a creative semi-nonfiction technique of rearranging a story's elements in order
to imagine or reimagine alternatives to historical accounts and give voice
to oppressed peoples whose stories are rarely told firsthand.

Bibliography

Alexander, M. Jacqui. 2005. *Pedagogies of Crossing: Meditations on Feminism,
Sexual Politics, Memory, and the Sacred.* Perverse Modernities. Durham,
NC: Duke University Press.

Allen, Jafari S., and Omise'eke Natasha Tinsley. 2012. "A Conversation 'Overflowing with Memory': On Omise'eke Natasha Tinsley's 'Water, Shoulders, into
the Black Pacific.'" *GLQ: A Journal of Lesbian and Gay Studies* 18, no. 2–3
(June): 249–62. https://doi.org/10.1215/10642684-1472881.

Boyce-Davies, Carole. 1994. *Black Women, Writing and Identity.* Oxford, U.K.:
Routledge.

——. 2013. *Caribbean Spaces: Escapes from Twilight Zones.* Urbana: University
of Illinois Press.

brown, adrienne maree. 2019. *Pleasure Activism: The Politics of Feeling Good.*
Emergent Strategy. Chico, CA: AK Press.

Brown, Khytie K. 2017. "The Spirit of Dancehall: Embodying a New *Nomos*
in Jamaica." *Transition*, no. 125: 17–31. https://muse.jhu.edu/article/686008.

Burleigh, Nina. 2020. "The Caribbean Dilemma." *New York Times*, August 4,
2020. https://www.nytimes.com/2020/08/04/travel/coronavirus-caribbean
-vacations.html.

Calypso Rose. 2016. "Leave Me Alone." Track 3 on Calypso Rose, *Far from
Home.* Maturity Music Ltd. / Stonetree Music Inc, compact disc.

Charles, Jacqueline, and Alex Harris. 2020. "Caribbean Nations Fighting
COVID-19 Blocked by Trump Policy." *Miami Herald*, April 13, 2020. https://
www.miamiherald.com/news/nation-world/world/americas/haiti/article
241922071.html.

Christopher, Peter. "Report on Police Killings in Morvant Sent to DPP." *Trinidad Guardian*, November 13, 2020. https://guardian.co.tt/news/report-on
-police-killings-in-morvant-sent-to-dpp-6.2.1250230.9f77c2e645.

Cowger, Tori L., Brigette A. Davis, Onisha S. Etkins, Keletso Makofane, Jour-
dyn A. Lawrence, Mary T. Bassett, and Nancy Krieger. 2020. "Comparison
of Weighted and Unweighted Population Data to Assess Inequities in Coronavirus Disease 2019 Deaths by Race/Ethnicity Reported by the US Centers

for Disease Control and Prevention." *JAMA Network Open* 3, no. 7 (July): e2016933. https://doi.org/10.1001/jamanetworkopen.2020.16933.

Davinchi, Zymora. 2020. "From #BlackLivesMatter to #VidasNegrasImportam: Call to End Colonial Legacy of Police Brutality." *Global Voices*, November 27, 2020. https://globalvoices.org/2020/11/27/from-blacklivesmatter-to -vidasnegrasimportam-call-to-end-colonial-legacy-of-police-brutality/.

Diamond, Dan. 2020. "'We Want Them Infected': Trump Appointee Demanded 'Herd Immunity' Strategy, Emails Reveal." *POLITICO*, December 16, 2020. https://www.politico.com/news/2020/12/16/trump-appointee-demanded -herd-immunity-strategy-446408.

Dutta, Sumita. 2016. "Spirits in the Food: A Pedagogy for Cooking and Healing." Master's thesis, Georgia State University. https://doi.org/10.57709 /8696135.

Gill, Lyndon K. 2018. *Erotic Islands*. Durham, NC: Duke University Press.

Goffe, Tao Leigh. 2019. "Sugarwork: The Gastropoetics of Afro-Asia After the Plantation." *Asian Diasporic Visual Cultures and the Americas* 51, no. 1–2 (April): 31–56. https://doi.org/10.1163/23523085-00501003.

Hartman, Saidiya V. 2008. "Venus in Two Acts." *Small Axe: A Caribbean Journal of Criticism* 12, no. 2 (June): 1–14. https://doi.org/10.1215/-12-2-1.

Henry, Onika. 2019. "Reclaiming Sexual Identity Through Carnival." TEDx Talks. Filmed November 25, 2019, in Port of Spain, Trinidad. YouTube video, 13:48. https://www.youtube.com/watch?v=uFn98nZnhCo.

IOM (International Organization for Migration). 2021. *Diaspora Groups of the Eastern Caribbean: Opportunities, Challenges and Needs for Collaboration*. San José, Costa Rica: IOM. https://kmhub.iom.int/sites/default/files/publi caciones/eastern_caribbean_diaspora_organization_mapping_final.pdf.

Jones, Kenneth, and Tema Okun. 2001. *Dismantling Racism: A Workbook for Social Change Groups*. N.p.: ChangeWork. https://www.dismantlingracism .org.

Liscia, Valentina Di. 2020. "As Brazil Grapples with Police Brutality, #Black-LivesMatter Murals Emerge in São Paulo." *Hyperallergic*, December 1, 2020. https://hyperallergic.com/604501/as-brazil-grapples-with-police-brutality -blacklivesmatter-murals-emerge-in-sao-paulo/.

Loop News. 2020. "Ornella Greaves Laid to Rest as Investigation Continues." July 8, 2020. http://www.looptt.com/content/ornella-greaves-laid-rest-investi gation-continues.

Lorde, Audre. 1978. *Uses of the Erotic: The Erotic as Power*. Brooklyn, NY: Out and Out Books.

———. 1982. *Zami: A New Spelling of My Name.* Crossing Press Feminist Series. Trumansburg, NY: Crossing Press.

Lorde, Audre, and Pat Parker. 2018. *Sister Love: The Letters of Audre Lorde and Pat Parker 1974–1989.* Edited by Julie R. Enszer and with an introduction by Mecca Jamilah Sullivan. Dover, FL: A Midsummer Night's Press.

Macoloo, Chris. 2020. "The Cultural and Social Challenges to Slowing the Pandemic in Africa." *Stanford Social Innovation Review,* May 8, 2020. https://ssir.org/articles/entry/the_cultural_and_social_challenges_to_slowing_the_pandemic_in_africa.

Moore, John. 2018. "They Travel with So Much: QandA with Monique Bedasse." *The Ampersand,* March 1, 2018. https://artsci.wustl.edu/ampersand/they-travel-so-much-qa-monique-bedasse.

Nap Ministry (@thenapministry). 2020. "How can we access pleasure & joy & liberation if we're too tired to experience it?" Instagram photo, June 10, 2020. https://www.instagram.com/p/CBQsrkBJyRD/.

Nixon, Angelique V. 2015. *Resisting Paradise: Tourism, Diaspora, and Sexuality in Caribbean Culture.* Jackson: University Press of Mississippi.

Osakwe, Chinekwu. 2020. "After Weeks of Protests, #EndSARS Has Become a Rallying Cry for a New Nigerian Generation." *Rolling Stone,* November 3, 2020. https://www.rollingstone.com/culture/culture-news/endsars-nigeria-davido-seun-kuti-1085353/.

Pate, Durrant. 2020. "US Warns Jamaica Against Chinese 5G." *Jamaica Observer,* October 25, 2020. https://www.jamaicaobserver.com/news/us-warns-jamaica-against-chinese-5g/.

Powerful, Sherine Andreine, Jallicia A. Jolly, and Kat Stephens. 2020. "Thriving Despite, Worlds-Shifting Through Corona." *Intersect Antigua,* October 31, 2020. https://www.intersectantigua.com/blog/thriving-despite-worlds-shifting-through-corona.

Steuart, Jada. 2020. "Black Lives Matter Protests in Trinidad and Tobago Spark Discussions About Race." *Global Voices,* June 9, 2020. https://globalvoices.org/2020/06/09/black-lives-matter-protests-in-trinidad-tobago-spark-discussions-about-race/.

Sutherland, Patsy, Roy Moodley, Barry Chevannes, and Pauletta Chevannes. 2013. *Caribbean Healing Traditions.* London: Routledge.

Tuck, Eve. 2009. "Suspending Damage: A Letter to Communities." *Harvard Educational Review* 79, no. 3 (Fall): 409–28. https://psycnet.apa.org/doi/10.17763/haer.79.3.n0016675661t3n15.

Washington Post. 2017. "'Reclaiming My Time': Rep. Maxine Waters Interrupts Mnuchin's Roundabout Answer." August 1, 2017. https://www.washington post.com/video/national/maxine-waters-reclaiming-my-time/2017/08/01 /30fae7f4-76d4-11e7-8c17-533c52b2f014_video.html.

Wormsley, Alisha B. n.d. There Are Black People in the Future. Accessed June 20, 2022. https://www.thereareblackpeopleinthefuture.com/.

Yosso, Tara J. 2005. "Whose Culture Has Capital? A Critical Race Theory Discussion of Community Cultural Wealth." *Race, Ethnicity and Education* 8, no. 1 (March): 69–91. https://doi.org/10.1080/1361332052000341006.

Femme Mixing

On an Erotics of Slowness and Its Wet Futures

Endia Hayes

Femme mixing[1] made itself known at the shared axes of searching for pleasure, my outpouring of lament, and my anger as I grappled with what I lost to the chaos of Ms. 'Rona, a colloquial term for COVID-19. At this time, *femme mixing* was my investment in the viscosity of what Lorde argues occurs when we do not, and perhaps cannot, turn from terror and unrest: we embrace the chaos of those axes of pleasure, lament, and anger, "which is Black which is creative which is fe[mme] which is dark which is rejected which is *messy*" (quoted in Morris 2002, 177). Thus with *femme mixing*, I name my personal, but more importantly, our shared messy slippages toward alternative temporal futures now rooted under the im/possibilities of slowness. In this essay, slowness is a tempo of Black femme futures, futures realized within the shifts of 2020, and what feels like heightened sense of precarity and unpredictable dangers. As I theorize around slowness, I present the "p(l)ace" of erotics tied to Black femme messiness across the U.S. South and beyond (Adeyemi 2019, 550).

Using the erotics of slowness prominent in 2020 *femme mixing*, I attend to how Black women and femmes express, and listen to, the gatherings of our innermost selves as sound and time drags. Meaning, as we believe that our fluctuations from crying to anger, from relief to sitting in the dark binging Netflix or social media, have felt lonely, we have in fact never been alone. Rather, forced isolation was just an uncovering of an erotic life under slowness. If we read 2020 and its continued reverberations like felt loss of time, as a slow tempo, Black femmes engage slowness as an erotic reinvestment in our lives in ways "align[ed] where and how we feel, where and how and who we love, where and how and whom we fuck" (Roach 2020, 180). Following Lorde's call to embrace the slipperiness of an erotic life, as well as Black feminisms' larger theorizing of knowing that rests in our flesh, slowness is an analytic through which we observed, participated, and embodied an imaginative sense of Black femme pace in 2020. This messy work of *femme mixing* both notes the violences ushered in by the COVID-19 pandemic and highlights the nonlinear, anticapitalistic, and wet work of Black women and femmes' slowly crafted futures.

Looking to Megan Thee Stallion's life and selections from her catalog as symbols of this *femme mix* under an erotics of slowness, I take examples from the Dirty South—a geography focused around a pace and aesthetic that has always moved against normal, against the fast-paced productivity of the assumed busyness of the North. It is this regional genealogy of slowness that superseded the pandemic and thus became layered under it; 2020 was thus slow tempo's event. As we witnessed, the U.S. South and Midwest were slow to a point of stagnation in responding to COVID, refusing to issue or enforce statewide shutdowns and mask requirements, and disregarding police brutality and accompanying protests. I ask how slowness calls us into futures that celebrate nonlinearity and the multidimensional creation of self. Drawing from southern sonic geographies, I prioritize a Black Texan femme sound that remains uncharted intellectual territory beyond Beyoncé yet has nurtured slowness in living and sound since the nineteenth century. These obfuscated interstices within Texas are fruitful enough for Megan to emerge leading this work and to, therefore, theorize the Black femme futures occurring in concert with slowness.

Mixing from the work of Black feminisms in hip-hop, and queer theory, I analyze the language used by Megan Thee Stallion under chopped and screwed sounds that signal how Black women and femmes have grappled with the 2020 pandemic—or the slow tempo of 2020. Megan Thee Stallion and her collaborators produce lyrics and imagery of wet(ness) either through ice, as in the slipperiness of affect in the song "Crying in the Car (Chopnotslop Remix)" from her *Suga (Chopnotslop) Remix* album, or through the use of *wet* to denote collective Black femme release under new temporalities—like Demon Time, in "Savage (Remix)" featuring Beyoncé and "WAP" with Cardi B. These examples of erotics under slowness occurring in popular music in 2020 are where Black women and femmes embraced the chaos of our innermost selves as both individual journeys and collective gatherings. Engaging these inner selves, often by indulging in bodily memory's liquid overflow, allows one to craft space expansive enough to experience release. This release is found in the anarchy of slow tempos and drawls of a Dirty South sonic geography, where 2020, and its impending afterlives, are disrupted by imaginative and sensorial space-times. Considering the potentials of slowness as a sonically located space, a visceral lyric, and a feel toward the fleshy excess of Black women and femme joy, *femme mixing* embraces the existence of futures that emerge otherwise. It makes space, creates a void—a sonic loophole of escape. It is the wet overflow of tears or c(u)m(m)ing under Demon Time that resonates throughout Megan's sonic mapping of survival; this is 2020's *femme mixing*.

Theorizing Black Femme Slowness, Its Erotics, and Its Possibilities

I begin with why looking to and with wet(ness) as an example of slowness's erotics in 2020's *femme mixing* advances key concepts located in the works of Black queer feminisms, Black feminist sex studies, and hip-hop feminisms.

Slowness sensually frames the time of release for Black femme erotic praxes. Slowness, here, is one provocative and sensuous quality of temporality underneath Black women and femmes' epistemologies created under the COVID pandemic. It is a knowing birthed from sensual freedom that—languidly, unhurriedly, gently, faster, taking time—embraces our chaotic attempts to define a life beyond 2020 death and its desired grabs for Black bodies. I use *wet(ness)* to denote the glissade of trial and error, success and improvement, struggle and excitement all associated with the violent ties of Black femme flesh to U.S. heteropatriarchal racial power. Clasping on to chaos as an invitation to become acquainted with the saturated portion of Black femme life undefined, this essay engages the quality and characteristics of wet(ness) to exhibit other temporal lifeworlds found in slowness. Following a genealogy of the erotic and its relations to slowness, and thus the wet, wet(ness) take three forms: icy affect, Demon Time, and sticky excess. Slowness does not in any way make 2020 a spectacular event. Rather, a turn to slowness is a turn to the interior drawls, and distorted tempos marked an unprecedented yet continued period of losses.

Reading Erotics Post-2020

In May 2020, I ended my semester earnestly revisiting and annotating Audre Lorde's (1984) pivotal text "Uses of the Erotic." Perhaps it was the social moment or the fact it was my third rereading in the past week, but what I found reoriented my perspective of erotics. Undergirding Lorde's lens of seeing and doing the work of erotics is mess. By *mess* I mean that under Black feminisms, locating and prioritizing desire is slippery, and, overall, a bit chaotic. This chaos, given that the Black femme lies at the crux of violence and endless possibility, alludes to a much larger experience that Lorde invites Black women and femmes into. By taking up this invitation, I reflected on the possible role of something akin to chaos as desirable under the conditions of 2020. In Lorde's legacy, Black feminisms are well acquainted with playing in this chaotic grabbing of a living futurity. It is the slowly revolving messiness of grabbing "living in a fundamental way" that materially and imaginatively builds on what Lorde, in interview with Claudia Tate, states must be developed "within ourselves," our "deepest life force" (1983, 115). Working from Lorde's perspective, I describe this as the innermost self of the femme, where our mutual searches for "the satisfying" meet (Lorde 1984, 59). Here, *mess* and *chaos*, if not synonymous, are foundational to Black *femme mixing*'s honoring of an interiority cultivated in what I am terming the "erotics of slowness," best defined as the chaotic slippage of Black femme possibilities. The erotics of slowness takes cues from Black queer feminisms, where attention to the sense(s) of the Black body serves as the location of pleasure and change.

Lorde (1984) maps the erotic's messiness as a micro (individual) to macro (communal) Black femme gathering. She begins by stating that to brush against life is to confront its strains, often by reconciling the tensions between us (Black women and femmes of the Diaspora) and intricate forms of oppression. We can define "reconciling" here as Lorde's way of foreshadowing the tangible expressions of knowing our innermost selves. Reconciling is no longer understood as settling but rather as a "radical praxis of politicizing the personal" (Roach 2020, 180). It is an ongoing recognition of where we lie in our relations and honoring our many attempts to move within and beyond them. Lorde reminds us that our work of knowing and expressing that inner self should never be done alone, but always in concert with others. This is Lorde's second point of the erotic—sitting with the ongoing collective of many individual expressions of discovered selves, a gathering of femme-inity "toward pursu[ing] genuine change" (1984, 59). It is important to note this gathering is a space without location, as we were reminded that we could not rely on a place like home (say her name, Breonna Taylor). Kemi Adeyemi reminds us that tempo and space are interwoven so much so that they redefine the "p(l)ace[s] of black people" (2019, 550). We can then think through Lorde's erotics

and an erotics of slowness as examples of the entanglements femme
bodies asks us to consider.

Black feminists who queer and theorize at the site of the innermost self begin with the confirmation of "what we know: our feelings"
(Roach 2020, 181); this is where we find joy. Across a "sharing of joy,"
discussions around the slipperiness of erotics for Black femme-inity,
or, as Lorde writes, "the beginnings of our sense of self and the chaos
of our strongest feelings" (1984, 54), start with the raunchy, the sexual, and, what I add, the wet. Focusing on the intersections between
body, sense, and mess, conversations on Black women and femme
erotics locate them at the disorderly slipperiness of encountering
both the resistant self and finding others who are, in fact, sensing this
p(l)ace, this future, with you. The Black femme body in (a) sense is, as
Aria Halliday states, the "epistemological imperative [of] the future"
(2020, 1). However we feel through various sites of chaotic encounter,
our moving and sensing through it is materially and imaginatively
"untidy" (McKittrick 2011, 949–51). Taking up the untidiness that
surrounds Black flesh—our "praxis and theory, [our] text for living
and for dying, and [our] method for reading both through their diverse mediations" (Spillers 1987, 68)—is to feel all of its fleshiness,
the inseparable "processes of objectification and the production of
selfhood" at the "limitlessness of insatiability" (Musser 2018, 1–2, 5).
The uncovering of "the satisfying" puts forward a variety of sensing
and knowing not only found at the gathering of a twerk but in Black
queer feminisms' fleshy concepts such as Black pussy power (Roach
2017), funk (Stallings 2015), and, what this essay advances, wet(ness) as
overflowing "bodily memory" (Tinsley 2008; Alexander 2005; brown
2019). The legacies of Lorde's erotic reveal the varied Black femme epistemologies emerging from "chaos" that are sensed (or known), and
located, on and outside the body. An erotics of slowness sits with the
possibilities that we have yet to fully make sense of what "produce[s]
experiential knowledge about the world" and that, in our gathering,

"'we' remain unexplored" (Halliday 2020, 877; Reed 2017, 23). The wet has little to no control when fully released. Wet(ness), the state and condition of being wet, actualizes the sloppiness of erotics.

Within an innermost self emerging under slowness, there is not only a noticeable temporal, corporeal, and vernacular shift but also sound and liquidity that convey how chaos is known and felt in Black femme-inity. Attending to the liquidity from this part of the Dirty South—an everyday naming of the unique Black southern culture prominently crafted under southern hip-hop—means tracing the affective, locative, and experiential (Williams 2018, 722) nature of slowness. One example L. H. Stallings provides of this is the aesthetics of slowness coming out of the Dirty South's drawls and slow tongues, praxes I pinpoint as also originating within the mess of Lorde's erotic. Slowness, therefore, invites an intimacy on "how to approach the dangers, fears, pleasures, and controversies that arise . . . [via] coax[ing] the listener's ear" (Stallings 2020, 22, 24). Stallings shows Black femme erotics as an integral part of a geographically and sonically locative interiority of Black southern life. Similarly, I see the Dirty South as a Black queer geography archived by sounds, sounds known because of their encounters with sensing, and therefore embodying, the desires of our innermost self.

Stallings (2020) continues rereading southern erotics through Houston's own "chopped and screwed" rap legacy, noting Millie Jackson as the erotic vocality that has defined this rap subgenre. Following in the style of Jackson's natural vocal manipulation that has crafted slowness as erotic storytelling, Stallings revises chopped and screwed genealogies by associating its foundations with Black femme sonic mapping between slowness and erotics in the mouth of Millie Jackson. Jackson, for instance, created texture with her voice, but it was manipulated by her producers as the depth of her voice was "too low for a woman" (Stallings 2020, 21). Jackson used her voice to give her listeners "natural," "lowered," and "husky" slow drawls reflective of seductive sex, foreplay, and an (over)abundance of erotic pleasure (21–22). A Black queer feminist approach to the erotics of slowness identifies a slipping between and sensing of the innermost self, imagining us within and wrestling with how we move through social, cultural, and even gendered tensions. These "slow tongues," as Stallings describes, "attend to form and aesthetics" that "will not only save your life [but] will make the life saved worth living" (17–18). Perhaps within the intimacy of slowness lies a mapping of the erotics that we need to save our lives.

Moving forward, this essay takes up lyrical themes around wet(ness) as a way of investigating the erotics of slowness exemplified in Megan Thee Stallion's music. I will often describe these themes in various ways, such as sticky excess, to name the multiple contexts in which the erotics of slowness shows up in Megan's lyrics. For example, sticky excess, or the visible extra-ness of wet(ness), denotes raunchy lyricism and imagery on and of the body, centering Black femme needs. I take up these themes, as charged by Black Dirty South feminist Adeerya Johnson, to focus on the language used by Black women and femmes in the stories they seek to tell in hip-hop (2019, 27). I argue that this language around *wet* speaks to the intersections between female hip-hop artists' making of futures navigated through erotics—and thus an erotics of slowness over the pandemic. *Wet*, as a vernacular shift, follows the slow choreographies of Black women and femme bodies as they lament unprecedented and sudden change, a lament that exists alongside messy grabs for the pleasure we deserve to release.

Black Femme and Wet Bodily Memory

Though I could spend time with the desire of Black masculinity that became the standard of slow storytelling in hip-hop, and in particular Houston's chopped and screwed genre, that is not the goal with this work. Instead, I am inspired by a conversation I had with Sherine Andreine Powerful and Onisha Etkins (2020) that fed this essay.[2]

Within our bodies lie all that we need: rememory, revolution from our ancestors, and intergenerational healing power poured out into our cooking, our rest, our dance—all indicators of how we as Black femmes of the Diaspora build the embodied archives of our lives. Drawing from the wisdom of Sherine, Onisha, and our Black feminist co-conspirators shared in text, laughter, and song over 2020–21, I observe a language of Black *femme mixing* from our flesh as we figure out, as we love, and as we find comfort in the chaos with which we take hold of the futures we slip into. Water's overflow touches our body's memories, often reverberations of the Atlantic (Alexander 2005; Allen and Tinsley 2012). But my interest in wet(ness) is an overflow from an erotics too long submerged to the point that when released, in rushes an excess of futures. The wet centers bodily release as a mode of re-centering Black femme-inity's range of living that never fully relied on any neoliberal understanding of normal but thrived on the strongest feelings that the erotics of slowness forces us to sit in.

"All of Them Nights That I Cried in the Car": Anger. Tears. Lament. Repeat.

It is important to note that Black women and femmes have felt too much. As the COVID pandemic has revealed the multilayered impacts of living under U.S. empire, a turn to slowness may feel like an exacerbation of the visceral felt condition of Black living during this time. Yet I want to position the im/possibility of this slipperiness as my sensing, or feeling, a future beyond this tumultuous period. I approach slipperiness from Megan Thee Stallion's demonstration that not all futures to be forged under slowness feel so easily attainable. Megan raps this slippery navigation of feeling, or what I will refer to as "icy affect" in "Crying in the Car (Chopnotslop Remix)." This song presents the affective possibilities that slowness makes space for, some of which were necessary in making sure that one, as an individual and in community, was all right. Through the lyrics, chopped and screwed tempo, and clear lyrical slippage between emotion, Thee MF Hot Girl tells a story of the very real instability of feeling that has occurred, continues to occur, and may eventually occur once more as Black women and femmes carry the weight of desiring radical futures for ourselves and our communities, all the while precariously remaining on the front lines.

Lament—worry, anger, unease, sadness, grief—as expressed through Megan Thee Stallion's (2020a) distorted raps in "Crying in the Car" adds to needed novelty around how and where Black femmes touch protection under the complex violences witnessed during the pandemic. She says,

People keep sayin' I should be the bigger person
Who's gonna worry 'bout me when I'm hurtin'?
Got one more time, keep talkin' that shit
And I'ma wild out and go hard on a bitch
I been stayin' up all night
My niggas in the street, I'm makin' sure they're alright

Megan is a protector and asserts herself as such. However, her want to protect appears affectively layered, and nonlinearly so. Hearing this tale in the slow feel of chop not slop, a listener may begin to feel the uncertainty and frustration of "Who's gonna worry 'bout me," which rises quickly, chaotically conflicted. In this stanza alone, Megan repeats her prayers, poignantly acknowledging that she cannot ignore the very imminent need/threat to care for herself as well as her "niggas in the street." Rather than questioning the weight that may come with ideas around Black women and femmes' responsibility in holding entire races and communities together at our own detriment, Megan feels the complicated affect that stems from an undecided, yet overwhelming, urgency to "mak[e] sure they're alright." Within the context of this complicated relation to everyone else except ourselves, several months later during her *Saturday Night Live* performance, Megan followed up with cries to "protect our Black women! And love our Black women! Because at the end of the day, we need our Black women!" (Megan Thee Stallion 2020c).

Megan pivots listeners toward the slipperiness, or this ice, of feeling. She asks that those impacted most by the un/wanted attention to Black femme life, and its value, freely slip through the waves of emotion felt throughout the pandemic—and sets up lament as "all of them nights that I cried in the car." This phrase laments what once was that quickly turned to abandonment. The uneasiness of crying for one's loneliness and one's niggas slips in and out of tension with violence present in our lives. Megan takes on icy affect, under slow tongues, expanding the conditions upon which Black femme futures expel slipperiness. In rejecting all sense of when and where to feel, Thee MF Hot Girl cries in the car as cathartic release to go "harder and harder"; she claims that "all them tears turned into ice on my arms." Despite Megan's reference to ice on her arms, under the erotics of slowness, I hesitate to read this statement as a turn to material wealth, even given the realities of inequitable living conditions. Rather, I focus on the messiness that causes ice to form in the first place. In its natural element, ice is not diamond watches or jewelry but the culmination of bonds, many of which are weak but rely on one another to form ice's physical properties. Perhaps ice, as element, forms in the continuation of our encounters with an event, a disaster, or stress, granting us even minimal opportunities to slip toward the bonds we hold. Regardless, Megan tells of affect's true reaction to Black femme-inity: it is slippery. As 2020's erotics of slowness has revealed, there lies an endless chaos of feeling—often leaving us with weak bonds and belief in a different global condition—but these affective oscillations have rarely been used to describe opportunity. What Megan submits to in "Crying in the Car" is the beauty of knowing that it is okay when we are not prepared for what comes next. Icy affect makes room. Those moments mark a free space to express our innermost (affective) selves slowly falling into tear-streaked cheeks and the taste of saltiness on our lips, described as messy, at best. Embracing icy affect calls Black women and femmes to keep "wild[in'] out" using that slipperiness off the heels of 2020's unpredictable scenes. Ice cuts through this lengthened violence, granting us room to mourn alone and in concert with others who are slipping on ice too.

Megan Thee Stallion (2020a) shares that slipping into icy affect under slowness occurs when

> I don't want to talk and I barely wanna listen
>
> . . . .
>
> I'm really happy that you muthafuckas hate me

Here, normal tempos and tongues no longer serve us—these tongues are steeped in anti-Blackness, LGBTQ+ and nonbinary phobia, and Black male patriarchy. Unlike the masculinity that sought ownership over the slow temporality of chopped and screwed traditions, what Black women and femmes throughout Texas's slow genealogies sought to protect through slowness was a bodily care running parallel to the violences of capitalism's demands. This is why we see mired response to Megan's own brush with violence from a Black male R & B artist, who will not receive the pleasure of being named in this essay. As anthropologist Nikki Lane (2021) writes, public responses to Megan Thee Stallion's shooting were conflicted, as the rapper was "ungrievable" because she is ratchet, or blatantly defiant of Black middle-class scripts of respectability (294). These responses are not new simply because of 2020. Instead what Megan contests through icy affect is an unapologetic refusal of the rapid disavowal of violence against Black women and femme life.[3] Icy affect signifies shifts in attitude, someone who under white capital's normal tempo is read as cold, unapproachable, or selfish, yet under slowness is unrepentantly embedded in their innermost self.

So, what does ice offer someone who seeks to give while needing care themselves? The answer to Megan's question "Who's gonna worry 'bout me when I'm hurtin'?" slips us into a wet quality of erotics of slowness that refuses a world that hates femme-inity. Here the slow tempos in Megan's *femme mixing* take characteristics of icy affect as a beyond where wet(ness) makes slipping out of capital, violence, and burden attainable.

When we center the types of drawls occurring in 2020 storytelling, slow tempos become a gateway to *femme mixes* that let Black women and femmes live in the beauty of the uncontrollability of icy, slippery affect. In light of Megan's intentional slow tempos, by chopping and *slipping* (not slopping), I next explore this culmination of wet excess for those of us gathering in these chaotic depths of slowness. Put simply, if we hold the futures made by Megan's attention to wet(ness) as fully accessible, then Black women and femmes may freely use slow tongues and tempos together.

The Sticky Excess of Demon Time, or We All Wet

Above Megan grapples with the liquidity in response to both her social environment and her personal desire to be present for herself and others. There is no balance where Megan's "Crying in the Car" is concerned. Instead, Megan exchanges balance for icy affect, or chaotic slipperiness, crying her way through uncertainty and fear. There is solace in the disorder of watery elements like ice and water, in mourning muddled pasts, the present, and futures. Yet even in thinking through ice, water's solid form, I sit with the use of wet(ness) that releases embodied memory. I consider how Megan's lyrics theorize wet(ness) not just as affective slippage but, in Lorde's (1984) second point about the erotic, as a map to collective femme community care, most notably in the collaborations "Savage (Remix)" featuring Beyoncé and "WAP" with Cardi B. "Savage (Remix)," I argue, attends to wet(ness) as an aesthetic of Black femme gathering under the erotics of slowness, presented as "Demon Time." Then, imagining within Demon Time, I again look at the form wet takes here. Next, though Megan references crying above as an entrance to feeling chaos, "WAP" uses *wet* as an example of the collective disruptions that sexual release of Black femme erotics under slowness delivers. Despite the song's heteronormativity, a focus on *wet* in "WAP" provides a queer outlook on suggestive gatherings of community care.

In "Savage (Remix)" (Megan Thee Stallion 2020d), Queen Bey calls to a different time of day, being, and performativity outside of normalcy, a call slowly drawing one into the erotics' seductive prospects.

Hips TikTok when I dance (dance)
On that Demon Time, she might start a OnlyFans (OnlyFans)

Thrusting listeners into this Demon Time builds on the indefinite chaos of slowness initiated by "Crying in the Car," one that relies on feeling, or perhaps slipping into, the mesmerizing sway of hips. Demon Time marks a chance to see what is not normally offered outside of it, hence Beyoncé's next lyrical tease: "If you wanna see some real ass, baby, here's your chance." This temporal erotic play—which under slowness speaks to further makings of Texas femme sonic geographies and the slow tempos that ran in tension to Texas governor Greg Abbott's push to remain in line with a "normal"—begins with "too much drip, ooh," an announcement of a wet(ness) that opens floodgates into Demon Time. Wanting to know what happens after dark, Demon Time mystifies why light is necessary in the first place when it truly does not change, and has not changed, the truths already revealed. Take, for example, Black women and femme lives that continue to sit at the forefront of police brutality, medical negligence, and racism, alongside gaslighting tactics challenging what we have seen and experienced in broad daylight and well-lit hospital rooms. Instead, from light we turn to a dark "Demon Time" where, deep inside a chaotic beyond, the gravity of our innermost selves pulls us into an unknown not directly seen. Instead, like Evelyn Hammonds (1994) suggests in "Black (W)holes and the Geometry of Black Female Sexuality," Black femme bodies possess the ability to consume, to draw in, to fully distort and disrupt all parts of normalcy. This slow, seducing consumption draws Black women and femmes in step with one another toward our self-cultivated digital, affective, and sonically embodied "p(l)aces." I pinpoint the use of Demon Time not to state that this is the only reading of welcoming the sensuality of darkness. Rather, Megan's call for Black femme listeners to consider darkness as the site of an indefinite erotics of slowness ("Bitch, what's happening?") points back to Black femme bodies as worthy to be consensually and safely seduced, desirable, and whole, an idea that Beyoncé reinforces:

I'm a bad *bitch*, she's a *savage*, no comparison here

....

Stallion when I ride him, like them hot girls, them hips, ah!

I hopped that shit, the way I hopped out and slid, ah! (emphasis

mine)

"Savage (Remix)" is a testament to living alone without ever being alone, holding space with others without being in proximity with them. Our desires are our pulls, and slips, into Demon Time. As Beyoncé vocalizes moving in and out, on and off, following Megan's "Ah," Beyoncé and Megan remain in constant conversation with each other. We hold so much drip, or wet(ness), that perhaps Demon Time feels like the sticky excess of the particular time and space that is *femme mixing*.

Further concretizing the sticky excesses of Demon Time, "WAP" utilizes *wet* to give us "something to believe in" (Cardi B 2020). Attending to ideas around the slipperiness of wet(ness), I move to conclude this essay by looking at what Roach calls "black pussy power," and rather than treating Black pussy as an object, one firmly held in heteronormativity, I point to the "W[et] A[ss] P[ussy]" power of sticky excess for "black fem[me-inity's] survival" (2017, 14). "WAP" highlights femme voices as authorities of their pleasure, and in the song's mission, a release, *a wet one*. Building on the sensual sonic practices of hip-hop's finest—such as Lil' Kim, Trina, Foxy Brown, and even Millie Jackson—and descriptions from disguises, wet beards, BDSM, cream, rides, and cum to that real wet macaroni sound when the loving gets good, "WAP" further places *femme mixing's* slow erotics as a sticky form of cleansing our sanctified w[ho(e)]lines:

Gobble me, swallow me, drip down the side of me

. . . .

I don't wanna spit, I wanna gulp

. . . .

Big D stand for big demeanor
I could make ya bust before I ever meet ya. (Cardi B 2020; all lines
   except second rapped by Megan Thee Stallion)

Sitting in, and on, the slipperiness of *wet*, the slow erotics of "WAP" vocalizes paths and promises of release. However, the song was met with great critique. With a focus on the slipperiness of the pussy and its slick characteristics that lead to release, wet(ness) refuses respectability, taking on the ecstasy of insuppressible c(u)m(m)ing under Demon Time. Wet(ness) heralds frequent climax and ultimate desire over the hesitation often projected on to Black women and femmes. In a *New York Times* article, Megan points to the backlash of not only "WAP" but her remorseless lyrical stance, stating that "when women choose to capitalize on our sexuality, to reclaim our *own* power, like I have, we are vilified and disrespected" (Megan

Thee Stallion 2020e). Therefore, we exercise wet(ness) and its Demon Time where we no longer carefully invested in pleasure-based
power.

Megan and Cardi B's particular attention to the lyrics and imagery
of the "wet" in "wet ass pussy" thrusts a flooding, or overwhelming,
imagery of an overflow of wet-based pleasure as one experiences a
sensually charged joy. Wet(ness) thus becomes an entrance for moving beyond just heteronormative desire. For example, womanist theo-
logian and essayist Candice Marie Benbow, after sharply critiquing
Black male responses to WAP's expressive claims to pleasure, tweeted
"*sages timeline and inbox with WAP*" (2020). It is this digital act of
cleansing that stems from the slow, sticky excesses within the song's
femme mixing. Our wet releases rid our futures of the toxins that expect our pleasure to be defined outside of our self and our community
of pleasure-seeking, pleasure-minded, pleasure-affirming erotic folks.
What "WAP" initiates, when read through wet(ness), speaks directly
against the rendering of Black women and femme flesh as lacking
and in need of saving from whitewashed ideas around sexuality, education, and spirituality, which are fueled by and exist alongside racist medical ideologies, a few white male trolls, and white feminism.
Wet(ness) sees a w[ho(e)]liness in celebration of the liquidity of our
innermost selves c(u)m(m)ing together. Sticky excess, using wet(ness)
as imagery for inviting in purifying power and energy, makes room
for femmes, as Megan puts it, to

Talk yo shit, bite yo lip
Ask for a car while you ride . . . (Cardi B 2020)

Demand, deny, expect, accept, and fuck, "coming into an aliveness
in your senses"—this is the space made under the slow tongues and
drawls of "WAP" (brown 2019, 121).

Yet, in response to the song's centering of the wet sanctification of Black women and femme pleasure under Demon Time, the white, male, settler, capitalist heteropatriarchy panicked. For example, Twitter quickly became overwhelmed by critiques from Republican politicians who wanted "to pour holy water in [their] ears" because the song was a result of "what happens when children are raised without God and without a strong father figure" (Paiella 2020). Ben Shapiro, founder of the *Daily Wire*, stated that to need "a bucket and a mop" required "medical care" because "[his] wife says that having a wet vagina is a medical condition . . . bacterial vaginosis, yeast infection, or trichomonas" (Paiella 2020). Under normal tempos, sharing sticky excess, especially in chorus with other femmes, is heavily racialized and sexualized. Black women and femme pleasure cannot exist without needing medical attention—it can only exist in defect. Once more, under normal tempos, sharing sticky excess, especially in concert with other femmes, is heavily racialized and sexualized. Vivid expressions of Black femme sexualities illustrated as unholy draw Black femmeinity into contestation with an idea of the divine. These deviant bodies lacking "father figure[s]" are then in need of patriarchal guidance to lead them back to the white lord's glory (Paiella 2020). Wet(ness) takes the Black femme body as w[ho(e)]ly, and thus has access to all the pleasure and excess hidden in the crevices of our bodily liquidity. It appeared as if Black men, white men, and white women remained uncomfortable with the visibility of an erotics of slowness so clearly public, particularly during a national and global crisis. It is no surprise then that the immediate backlash to "WAP" greatly contradicted the larger cries, social media campaigns, and protests for greater public support of Black women and femmes just a month or so earlier, ones Megan was vocal about.

"WAP" is a *femme mixed* conversation. Less than a month following Megan being shot by a male R & B artist, who will not receive the pleasure of being named here, Cardi B and Megan Thee Stallion demanded that their listeners take in the slow, sticky excesses of being able to be and feel wet—a quality shared across innermost selves. Both artists respond to the other, c(u)m(m)ing together to celebrate a shared found pleasure in an erotics of slowness. This conversation, homegirl to homegirl, already takes place in a future cultivated by the sticky excess of wet, slow tempos deep within Demon Time. Particularly, Megan and Cardi slow-tongue a life worth living beyond the edge. Here, to "gobble [femmes], swallow [femmes], drip down the side of [femmes]" plays on the ever-present future made by the pleasures and longevity of the wet(ness) of *femme mixing*.

sages [the readers of this essay] with WAP

Conclusion

On November 11, 2020, CNN named Texas the first state to have over 1 million COVID-19 cases (Maxouris 2020). This statement is not to portray Texas as an exception but rather to point out the unusual times that appear to only have gotten worse. I felt like I was losing a grasp on my reality: my family's well-being, my partner's and my celebration of new chapters, the overwhelming heaviness of consistent loss of life, and the realization that I was driving my inner self into overwhelming stagnation. Slowness felt like my enemy.

Simultaneously, in witnessing Megan Thee Stallion's *femme mixing*, I was provided with a blueprint, a more capacious outlook on these slow times, making complex, and pertinent, the futures accessible to Black women and femmes now. It is wet(ness) that grapples with the ever-slippery attempts to escape the reaches of the U.S. empire upon Black life, a living that never was normal. In the spirit of the good news that Megan and her collaborators bring, the messy wet(ness) of Black women and femme erotics of slowness attend to what Lorde names as the "yes within ourselves, [the yes of] our deepest cravings" (1984,

57). *Femme mixing* celebrates the necessity of slowness when centering the stories we often move too fast to attend to but are often forced to confront anyway; this is the power of Megan's 2020 sonic gift.

This essay is not to leave *femme mixing* in a monolithic category of understanding but to hopefully unravel the drawls of where I see erotics crucially emerging by and for Black women and femmes under the age of Ms. 'Rona. Though I depended heavily on how it emerges in the intimate entanglements between sonic geographies and its embodied praxes, the fleshy dis-ease that *femme mixing* brings is the only way forward, as seen in the riffs of Megan Thee Stallion's music and life. Megan raps to Lorde's "yes" and her "deepest cravings," stating that between her "stank ass walk" and "reckless ass mouth," she does not care; instead, she implores Black women and femmes, "don't stop" (Megan Thee Stallion 2020b). So it begins under all thangs wet—the sacredness of release, of tears, moaning, and cum. Sitting under *femme mixing*, these now-sacred praxes of indulging the chaos of our inner selves make space and, most importantly, make time for us to touch, feel, and lie in the erotics of slowness.

Notes

1. This essay's focus on *femme mixing* requires a brief note on how I am conceptualizing *femme*. *Femme*, here, builds from Jessica Marie Johnson's (2018) ode to what she titles "Black Femme Forms of Knowledge and Practice." The black femme, she states, "dissemble[s], dismantle[s] and seek[s] fragments of ourselves" (666). As Story articulates, femmes as both creators and makers of performance and identity dwell in a "resistive femininity" that shifts how they come to understand their intersections of race, gender, and sexuality (2017, 419). Thus, *femme* exhibits a being built on fluid femininity, practice, and erotic creation and performance.

2. This conversation—one of many we had over the course of 2020 and 2021—took place in a writing group with Sherine and Onisha. We focused on how to best write about joy, pleasure, and full femme-inity throughout the pandemic. The conversation I cite was one that particularly spoke to embodied ways of knowing—ways that stemmed from recipes, rituals,

and dance. We spoke of how much our movements, cooking, and life intimately connected and collected, breaking a space-time continuum. Our memories of joy were sacred, and they were readily accessible.

3. On July 12, 2020, Megan was shot by a popular male R & B artist, well known for his own use of sampling and remixes. After weeks of speculation following the release of an aerial helicopter video where an injured Megan limped from an SUV, reports eventually announced that Megan had been shot in both feet while attempting to exit the vehicle following an argument. Megan, after having surgery on both feet to remove bullet fragments, took her time addressing the event that took place. Eventually, she confirmed on an Instagram live, yelling, "[N]igga! . . . You shot me!" (Rindner 2022).

Bibliography

Adeyemi, Kemi. 2019. "The Practice of Slowness: Black Queer Women and the Right to the City." *GLQ: A Journal of Lesbian and Gay Studies* 25, no. 4 (October): 545–67. https://doi.org/10.1215/10642684-7767767.

Alexander, M. Jacqui. 2005. *Pedagogies of Crossing: Meditations on Feminism, Sexual Politics, Memory, and the Sacred*. Perverse Modernities. Durham, NC: Duke University Press.

Allen, Jafari S., and Omise'eke Natasha Tinsley. 2012. "A Conversation 'Overflowing with Memory': On Omise'eke Natasha Tinsley's 'Water, Shoulders, into the Black Pacific.'" *GLQ: A Journal of Lesbian and Gay Studies* 18, no. 2–3 (April): 249–62. https://doi.org/10.1215/10642684-1472881.

Benbow, Candice Marie (@candicebenbow). 2020. "*sages timeline and inbox with WAP*." Twitter, August 21, 2020. https://twitter.com/candicebenbow /status/1291736277080059905?s=21andt=SIVKXQ1B2i4bdtCh2WiMCg.

brown, adrienne maree. 2019. "Wherein I Write About Sex (Five Tangible Tools of a Pleasure Activist)." In *Pleasure Activism: The Politics of Feeling Good*, 96–103. Chico, CA: AK Press.

Cardi B. 2020. "WAP," featuring Megan Thee Stallion. Spotify, single released August 2020. Atlantic Records.

Halliday, Aria. 2020. "Twerk Sumn! Theorizing Black Girl Epistemology in the Body." *Cultural Studies* 34, no. 6 (January): 874–91. https://doi.org/10.1080 /09502386.2020.1714688.

Hammonds, Evelyn. 1994. "Black (W)holes and the Geometry of Black Female Sexuality." *Differences: A Journal of Feminist Cultural Studies* 6, no. 2–3 (Summer/Fall): 126–45. https://doi.org/10.1215/10407391-6-2-3-126.

Hartman, Saidiya. 2020. *Wayward Lives, Beautiful Experiments: Intimate Histories of Social Upheaval*. New York: W. W. Norton.

Johnson, Adeerya J. 2019. "Spill the Tea Sis': Misogynoir's Problem and Black Women's Support, Narratives and Identities Found in *Love and Hip-Hop*'s Reality TV Franchise." Master's thesis, Georgia State University. https://doi.org/10.57709/14694544.

Johnson, Jessica Marie. 2018. "4DH + 1 Black Code / Black Femme Forms of Knowledge and Practice." *American Quarterly* 70, no. 3 (September): 665–70. https://doi.org/10.1353/aq.2018.0050.

Lane, Nikki. 2021. "Ratchet Black Lives Matter: Megan Thee Stallion, Intra-Racial Violence, and the Elusion of Grief." *Linguistic Anthropology* 31, no. 2 (September): 293–97. https://doi.org/10.1111/jola.12323.

Lorde, Audre. 1984. "Uses of the Erotic: The Erotic as Power." In *Sister Outsider: Essays and Speeches*, 53–59. Crossing Press Feminist Series. Trumansburg, NY: Crossing Press.

Maxouris, Christina. 2020. "Texas Becomes the First US State with More Than 1 million COVID-19 Infections." CNN, November 11, 2020. https://www.cnn.com/2020/11/11/us/texas-one-million-covid-cases/index.html.

McKittrick, Katherine. 2011. "On Plantations, Prisons, and a Black Sense of Place." *Social and Cultural Geography* 12, no. 8 (October): 947–63. https://doi.org/10.1080/14649365.2011.624280.

Megan Thee Stallion. 2020a. "Crying in the Car (Chopnotslop Remix)." Spotify, track 8 on Megan Thee Stallion, *Suga (Chopnotslop Remix)*. 300 Entertainment.

———. 2020b. "Don't Stop," featuring Young Thug. Spotify, track 17 on Megan Thee Stallion, *Good News*. 300 Entertainment and 1501 Certified Entertainment.

———. 2020c. *Saturday Night Live*. Clip from season 46, episode 1, hosted by Chris Rock. Aired October 3, 2020, on NBC. YouTube video, 4:08. https://www.youtube.com/watch?v=CTpilDQXYr0.

———. 2020d. "Savage (Remix)," featuring Beyoncé. Spotify, single released April 2020. 300 Entertainment and 1501 Certified Entertainment.

———. 2020e. "Why I Speak Up for Black Women." *New York Times*, October 13, 2020. https://www.nytimes.com/2020/10/13/opinion/megan-thee-stallion-black-women.html.

Morris, Margaret Kissam. 2002. "Audre Lorde: Textual Authority and the Embodied Self." *Frontiers: A Journal of Women Studies* 23, no. 1: 168–88. https://doi.org/10.1353/fro.2002.0009.

Musser, Amber. 2018. *Sensual Excess: Queer Femininity and Brown Jouissance.* New York: New York University Press.

Paiella, Gabrielle. 2020. "Wait, What: The Week in 'WAP.'" *GQ*, August 14, 2020. https://www.gq.com/story/the-week-in-wap.

Rearick, Lauren. 2020. "Beyoncé and Megan Thee Stallion Drop 'Savage' Remix with Proceeds for Charity." *Teen Vogue*, April 29, 2020. https://www.teen vogue.com/story/beyonce-megan-thee-stallion-savage-remix-charity.

Reed, Anthony. 2017. "The Erotics of Mourning in Recent Experimental Black Poetry." *Black Scholar* 47, no. 1 (January): 23–37. https://doi.org/10.1080/000 64246.2017.1264851.

Rindner, Grant. "Megan Thee Stallion on Shooting Skeptics: 'I'm the Victim.'" *GQ*, April 25, 2022. https://bit.ly/3AaHwVM.

Roach, Shoniqua. 2017. "Black Pussy Power: Performing Acts of Black Eroticism in Pam Grier's Blaxploitation Films." *Feminist Theory* 19, no. 1 (December): 7–22. https://doi.org/10.1177%2F1464700117742866.

———. 2020. "On the Uses of Black Feminism: Notes on Black Feminism as Sexuality Study." *Feminist Formations* 32, no. 1 (Spring): 180–88. http://doi .org/10.1353/ff.2020.0015.

Spillers, Hortense. 1987. "Mama's Baby, Papa's Maybe: An American Grammar Book." *Diacritics* 17, no. 2 (Summer): 64–81. https://doi.org/10.2307/464747.

Stallings, L. H. 2015. *Funk the Erotic: Transaesthetics and Black Sexual Cultures.* Chicago: University of Illinois Press.

———. 2020. *A Dirty South Manifesto: Sexual Resistance and Imagination in the New South.* Oakland: University of California Press.

Story, Kaila Adia. 2017. "Fear of a Black Femme: The Existential Conundrum of Embodying a Black Femme Identity While Being a Professor of Black, Queer, and Feminist Studies." *Journal of Lesbian Studies* 21, no. 4 (October): 407–19. https://doi.org/10.1080/10894160.2016.1165043.

Tate, Claudia, ed. 1983. "Audre Lorde." In *Black Women Writers at Work*, 100–116. New York: Continuum Publishing.

Tinsley, Omise'eke Natasha. 2008. "Black Atlantic, Queer Atlantic: Queer Imaginings of the Middle Passage." *GLQ: A Journal of Lesbian and Gay Studies* 14, no. 2–3: 191–215. https://doi.org/10.1215/10642684-2007-030.

Williams, Rhaisa Kameela. 2018. "Choreographies of the Ongoing: Episodes of Black Life, Events of Black Lives." *Biography* 41, no. 4 (Fall): 760–76. https:// doi.org/10.1353/bio.2018.0078.

CHAPTER 3

Black Women and Coronavirus in the United Kingdom

The Need for a Black Feminist Epidemiology

Jenny Douglas

Introduction

As the extent and reach of coronavirus emerged globally, one of my first thoughts was about how other Black women had experienced and survived such pandemics in the past. I searched the literature for the experiences of Black women in the United Kingdom during the 1918–19 influenza pandemic. Not only could I not find any accounts or narratives written by Black women, but it appeared that although there has been a Black presence in Britain since Roman times (Fryer 2018) and there were Black communities in the United Kingdom in 1918, they had been written out of history. Green (1998) argues that although Black people were active in many places and in many ways in early twentieth-century Britain, evidence of their presence was scattered and not documented in mainstream history books. In *Black Poppies: Britain's Black Community and the Great War*, Stephen Bourne (2019) documents the experiences of some Black servicemen and the wider Black community in Britain from 1914 to 1919. Bourne makes scant reference to Black women, aside from noting that Black women had limited career choices during the First World War and that although there was a "need for hospital and Red Cross nurses during the First World War, there is no evidence that any black woman was given the opportunity to join the nursing profession"

(Bourne 2019, 167). Furthermore, research undertaken into the role of women in the First World War concluded that there was no documentary or photographic evidence of Black women nursing in the United Kingdom's civil hospitals or military hospitals (Bourne 2019). Black Caribbean women were not recruited to the Women's Auxiliary Air Force or the Auxiliary Territorial Service until the Second World War, and not until 1943 (Bourne 2018).

Hence, there was very little documented about the experiences of Black women in the United Kingdom in 1918, and in the emerging literature on Black British history, Black women were to a large extent invisible. I then searched the literature to explore how Black women in the United States experienced the 1918–19 influenza pandemic. Again, I could not find any accounts or direct narratives written by Black women. However, I discovered that Nella Larsen, an African American novelist of the Harlem Renaissance, had been a public health nurse during the influenza pandemic, working for the city Bureau of Public Health in the Bronx (Hutchinson 2006). Nella Larsen published two novels: *Quicksand* (1928) and *Passing* (1929). *Quicksand* was thought to be largely autobiographical and focused on racial identity and experiences of African Americans in Harlem, and so Larsen may have drawn on her experiences working as a nurse in an agency that was at the cutting edge of public health in June 1918, just as the influenza epidemic was taking hold of New York City. Her second novel, *Passing*, focused on racial passing—the attempts by some Black people to "pass" as white—and also presented a critical analysis of race, gender, and sexuality. It is possible that her experience as a public health nurse living and working in Harlem through a global pandemic also contributed to this novel.

Nella Larsen's work and the employment experiences of other African American nurses demonstrate the ways in which Black women were seen as a reserve army of labor—pulled in when needed to do jobs that white women would not want to do and then discriminated against and excluded when they weren't needed. Although Black hospitals and hospital-based nurse training programs were established between 1891 and 1907, and the 1910 census recorded 3,100 Black women nurses (Jones and Saines 2019), Black women were denied employment in mainstream (segregated) hospitals and organizations and barred from membership in the American Nurses Association (Hine, 1989). Many Black nurses applied to work in the 1914–18 war effort but they were excluded from wartime military service in the American Red Cross, the U.S. Army Nurse Corps, and the U.S. Navy Nurse Corps (Jones and Saines 2019). Being unable to serve in the war effort, they were also denied the benefits that white nurse veterans received when the war ended in November 1918. However, when the pandemic peaked in November 1918, so did the demand for Black nurses.

Larsen was one of many African American nurses employed during the 1918–19 influenza pandemic and her experience as a public health nurse reveals the history of discrimination and exclusion widely experienced by Black nurses in the United States at this time. The pandemic provided the opportunity for African American nurses to go into homes of people who were sick and dying—which made for difficult, dangerous work. African American nurses like Larsen were put on twelve-hour shifts seven days a week when the second wave of the pandemic occurred in the autumn of 1919. As Hutchinson recounts, "Larsen worked seven days a week, with little sleep. The work was harrowing. A nurse might enter a stinking apartment to find both parents dead, or children dead and parents too sick to know it" (2006, 119).

Despite the brutal work, there were no reported deaths of Black nurses during this pandemic; however, there was little systematic data collection, so this is not conclusive. And once the pandemic was over, Black women once more continued to experience racism and discrimination in obtaining positions as nurses.

The raced, classed, and gendered position of Black women in the United Kingdom and the United States has rendered them invisible in mainstream historical accounts. They are only noteworthy when they are employed in particular professions—as nurses, for example. I have chosen to articulate the position of Black women nurses, as we have data on their employment, which we do not have for all other Black women at the turn of the twentieth century. There is also data, albeit patchy and inconclusive, on Black women in the armed forces in both the First and Second World Wars. These data, although incomplete, demonstrate that Black women experienced discrimination in employment both in the armed forces in the United Kingdom and United States and in nursing in the two jurisdictions. The lack of data in employment has a greater significance in relation to health and the incidence of particular conditions and illnesses. In order to develop appropriate health promotion and health protective services, there must be relevant and appropriate data. This essay outlines the need to develop methodologies that collect, document, and analyze the health experiences of Black women.

COVID-19 and Black Women in the United Kingdom: An Overview

The severity of the COVID-19 pandemic in the United Kingdom became a major concern to politicians and policy makers in March 2020. The prime minister announced the first lockdown on March 23, 2020, and people were ordered to "stay at home." Although the lockdown was lifted on July 4, 2020, further local lockdowns were subsequently introduced in areas of England, such as parts of Leicestershire, because of soaring levels of COVID-19. It was interesting that these areas had substantial Black and other minority ethnic populations, and this may have influenced the decision for further lockdowns. An initial report by the Office for National Statistics (ONS) that examined COVID-19-related deaths by ethnic group in England and Wales between March 2, 2020, and April 10, 2020, revealed that after adjusting for age, men and women from all ethnic minority groups (except females with Chinese ethnicity) were at greater risk of dying from COVID-19 compared with those of white ethnicity. As I will explain, the main reason for the higher incidence of COVID-19 in certain populations was through occupational exposure. For the Chinese ethnic group, the research reported a raised risk among males but not females (ONS 2020); later research demonstrated that Chinese females were less likely to be working in frontline occupations where they were exposed to COVID-19. Black males were 4.2 times more likely to die from COVID-19 than white males, while Black females were 4.3 times more likely to die from COVID-19 than white females, and people of Bangladeshi, Pakistani, Indian, and mixed ethnicities also had statistically significantly raised odds of death compared with those of white ethnicity (ONS 2020). At this point, Black women appeared to be the group that was most impacted by COVID-19, and ONS suggested that while this was partly due to socioeconomic disadvantage, the differences could not be fully explained. One of the limitations of the analysis was that ethnicity was not routinely recorded on the death certificate and hence the 2011 census was used to undertake an analysis using self-reported ethnicity and demographic factors of people who died. Public Health England (PHE 2020a) published a report after the ONS report based on an analysis of data between March 21 and May 1. In this analysis, Black males were 3.9 times more likely and Black females were 3.3 times more likely to die than white males and females, respectively, and PHE reported that this data was similar to the ONS (2020) data; we can see that although Black people are the most impacted group, in this analysis, Black men are more likely to be impacted when compared to Black women. Thus, we are starting to see differences and limitations in the epidemiological analyses undertaken. There was widespread criticism following the publication of the first PHE report, focusing on the fact that although Black and minority ethnic (BME) communities appeared to be at disproportionate risk of COVID-19, this report made no attempt to explain why this was the case; it seemed to be missing a substantive section informed by wide consultation with BME communities. The long-awaited second report (PHE 2020b) addressed earlier criticisms and put forward a complex interplay of structural, social, economic, political, and environmental explanations for the disproportionate disparities experienced by BME communities. In relation to BME health workers, the report highlighted that not only were these workers more likely to be frontline workers, and therefore at greater risk of acquiring COVID-19 infection, but because of structural racism that exists in organizations like the National Health Service (NHS) and transport services, BME workers were less able to express their concerns in workplaces where bullying, discrimination, and racism were rampant. Many BME people were key workers in the NHS, health and social services, transport services, and in housing. Their occupations required social contact, which put them at greater risk of being exposed to COVID-19. In addition, these key workers were required to go to work during the pandemic and often were using public transport themselves, which was another source of exposure. In the early days of the pandemic, many BME workers did not have appropriate personal protective equipment (PPE), and they often felt pressured to work longer hours than usual or than they were contracted to work (Ford 2020).

In addition to being at greater risk because of their jobs, for some BME communities, the neighborhoods where they lived, with dense housing, also increased the risk of exposure and infection. For example, intergenerational families living in cramped housing conditions did not allow space for required social isolation if COVID-19 was contracted by members of the family. "Overcrowded households among BME populations are also much more likely to be multigenerational, making social distancing, self-isolation and shielding much more difficult, and increasing opportunities for within-household coronavirus transmission" (Independent Sage 2020). Some authors have also pointed to the fact that BME people did not receive appropriate care or information from primary care services and were discriminated against by hospitals (Charity So White, n.d.). It was also argued that BME patients with COVID-19 fared worse in the development and progression of COVID-19 because they were more likely to have underlying health conditions such as diabetes, hypertension, and obesity, which led to a more severe COVID-19 infection. Many BME people were more likely to have existing comorbidities, multiple long-term conditions, chronic diseases, and also severe mental illness, and they experienced structural racism in access to and provision of health services (Gopal and Rao 2021). Thus, COVID-19 exacerbated existing long-standing, deep-rooted, persistent, and enduring health inequities already experienced by BME communities, inequities that were themselves due to structural factors such as racism, discrimination, and socioeconomic disadvantage (Godlee 2021). This was further compounded for Black women by sexism and the need to work for their economic security. There is a growing literature on the effects of racism and discrimination on the health and wellbeing of BME communities and the impact of this across people's life course (Douglas 2018), and this experience is mirrored in relation to the risk, exposure, and progression of COVID-19. From consultation with community organizations, PHE (2020b) concluded that based on previous negative experiences with health services and a lack of trust in NHS services, people from BME communities were less likely to seek opportunities for testing despite the wide availability and accessibility of testing sources and stations, and were also more likely to present late for treatment for the disease. Furthermore, the fear of death and stigma associated with COVID-19 led to late diagnosis even though there was access to local hospitals.

While COVID-19 has disproportionately affected the lives of all BME communities, Black women across the United Kingdom are more likely than their white female counterparts to have been hospitalized and/or died, for a variety of complex and interrelated reasons related to their classed, gendered, and racialized positions. A large number of Black women are employed in the NHS as nurses, health workers, auxiliaries, and cleaners. Black women were initially recruited from the Caribbean when the NHS was founded in 1948, and then later from Africa; they continued to be recruited through 1950s and 1960s, a period called the Windrush era, and are still significantly employed in health and social care. Black nurses felt that they were being targeted to work on COVID-19 wards and therefore being exposed to COVID patients over and above their white colleagues (Ford 2020). Because of prevailing racism and discrimination, many Black nurses felt that they were unable to discuss their concerns with their line managers or departmental managers (Douglas 2022; Bernard and Harewood 2021). Most Black women were working on the front line as nurses, social workers, and transport workers, and were not able to work from home. Transport workers, working in stations, such as bus drivers and taxi drivers, were also at greater risk of acquiring COVID-19 and often were not provided with appropriate PPE.

Thus Black women were at the greatest risk from COVID-19, and COVID-19 has exacerbated existing and long-standing inequities in health that have stemmed from structural racism in all aspects of their lives. The political context in which Black women live further extends inequities. One of the main drivers for Brexit, for example, was to reduce immigration of Black people. Black women in the United Kingdom currently live in a hostile environment that has been building for decades, notably demonstrated by the "Windrush betrayal" (Gentleman 2020): Some of the very women who were invited to work in the newly formed NHS in the mid-twentieth century were later denied their British citizenship, made unemployed, made homeless, and denied access to health and social care. Some people were arrested and placed in deportation centers and some were deported to the Caribbean. Following an investigation, a compensation scheme was established, but some of the Windrush scandal victims died before they received any compensation. A further, contemporary example of this hostile environment is the 2017 Grenfell Tower fire, which caused seventy-two deaths, with more than seventy other people injured. The fire was caused by flammable cladding applied to the exterior of the building. The majority of the residents in the tower were from BME communities and the subsequent inquiry concluded that the fire was inextricably linked with race (McKee 2017). The Windrush betrayal and the Grenfell Tower fire shone a light on the experiences of racism and discrimination experienced by Black people in the United Kingdom.

It is against this backdrop that I will outline the narratives of two Black women who died due to their occupational exposure to COVID-19. Belly Mujinga was a railway ticket office worker at Victoria Station in London (Campbell 2021). She had underlying health issues, and although she had informed her managers of this, she was required to work because of severe staff shortages. She was spat at by a member of the public, who said that he had COVID-19, on March 22, 2020. She and her colleague fell ill with COVID-19, and Mujinga died on April 5, 2020. Two years later, no one has been charged with any crime, as the Crown Prosecution Service concluded that there was insufficient evidence. Initially, there had been no investigation into her death, despite calls for a coroner's inquest by the union to which she belonged, the Transport Salaried Staffs' Association (TSSA). Following lobbying from the TSSA, the coroner decided to hold an inquest. Lawrence Davies, a solicitor for Mujinga's family, stated in a press release: "It will address the health and safety problems (lack of PPE) faced by frontline workers during the Covid pandemic; and particularly those with underlying health issues, as well as the racism and harassment that BME frontline workers face at work, and it will finally allow us to call to account the intemperate white male who the family alleges assaulted Mujinga and her colleague, Motolani, twice on the concourse of Victoria Station on 21 March 2020" (Campbell 2021). At the time of writing, the inquest has been delayed until summer 2022; a May 2022 news article reports that the inquest will not consider the spit attack, but rather will focus on whether Mujinga "should have been shielding at the time" (ITV News 2022).

Mary Agyeiwaa Agyapong, a pregnant hospital nurse, also died of COVID-19, and her baby daughter was delivered by an emergency caesarean section. She tested positive for COVID-19 on April 5, 2020, and died on April 7. Mary had worked until March 12 and was admitted to hospital with breathing problems on April 5, where despite the assessment that she was suspected to have COVID-19 and the fact that she was heavily pregnant, she was sent home because she did not appear to need oxygen. On April 7, Agyapong was then readmitted and died in intensive care on April 12. Mary had continued to work in the hospital because of the high demand for nurses and feeling pressured to work despite the worry for her own health. The coroner concluded that it was not clear where she had been exposed to the virus, as she had not been working for a few weeks before (between March 12 and April 5), and therefore she may not have acquired COVID-19 through occupational exposure at her workplace. Clinicians at the hospital where she worked had raised concerns about safety at work and the lack of PPE available to frontline staff (Slater and Fagge 2020).

These two cases demonstrate how their raced, classed, and gendered position placed Black women at greater risk of exposure to and death from COVID-19. Both Black women were at greater risk of exposure because of their employment as frontline workers; they were pressured to continue working, and because of their socioeconomic position and fears of losing their jobs, as well as their commitment to supporting the effort of their organization in combatting COVID-19, they continued to work in conditions that they considered unsafe and injurious to their health. Mujinga was exposed to racist abuse and Agyapong appears to have received poor treatment in the hospital. We can ask the question: Why was Agyapong sent home on April 5? In both instances, Black women were put at greater risk of occupational exposure to COVID-19.

There are enduring inequities in Black women's health and well-being in the United Kingdom, in relation to diabetes, hypertension, mental health, breast cancer, and maternal mortality and morbidity (Douglas 2018). A Maternal, Newborn and Infant Clinical Outcome Review Programme (MBRRACE-UK) report (2018) states that "there are striking inequalities: black women are five times and Asian women two times more likely to die as a result of complications in pregnancy than white women and urgent research and action to understand these disparities is needed" (Knight et al. 2018). Despite the recognition that urgent research is needed, there is still a gap in the public health evidence available to understand why Black women are at greater risk of maternal mortality. There is a need for research studies involving and led by Black women.

The health activism of Black women has largely been ignored by historians, sociologists, and white feminist scholars (Douglas 2019). However, despite the greater impact of COVID-19 on Black women, Black women have demonstrated their agency by creating and developing organizations that have supported Black communities throughout the pandemic and by providing relevant and appropriate public health information—such as how the virus is transmitted and the signs of infection. Organizations such as the Ubele Initiative and Caribbean and African Health Network have set up counseling services for people who have been bereaved by COVID-19; the Ubele Initiative has also established the Majonzi COVID-19 Bereavement Fund to provide support to BME community members who have lost loved ones to the disease. The grief that COVID-19 has caused to Black communities in the United Kingdom falls against the backdrop of the Windrush betrayal and Grenfell Tower disaster. Black women activists, despite their fear and grief, have developed online resources to raise awareness in Black communities about vaccination, providing hope and the necessary support and resilience to build better Black communities for the future. Research organizations and academic institutions still need to develop opportunities for Black women to lead research to develop epidemiological approaches and methodologies based on a Black feminist epistemology so that we can fully record, investigate, analyze, and understand the impact of COVID-19 on Black women. By developing appropriate, intersectional epidemiological approaches, the whole of society will benefit, and we will be better placed to respond effectively to the next pandemic.

Critique of Epidemiological Frameworks

Black women needed culturally relevant and appropriate information on COVID-19 and safe and accessible health services that ensure Black women do not experience racially discriminatory or disadvantageous treatment. The planning, design, and development of such health services require appropriate epidemiological data. Traditional epidemiological approaches can mask or hide the specific experiences of Black women. A Health Foundation report proposed that in interpreting research on ethnicity and COVID-19 risk and outcomes, five questions should be asked:

1. Does the report take into account the social context in which ethnicity is defined?
2. What explanations does the report give for differences between ethnic groups in risk and outcomes of COVID-19?
3. Are the analytical methods used appropriate for testing these explanations?
4. Does the report use appropriate data?
5. Who was consulted and what level of involvement did they have in the report?

(Stafford et al. 2020)

While this framework moves toward a more equitable epidemiological approach, further steps are required in order to develop a Black feminist approach to knowledge production and epidemiology.

Proposed Black Feminist Epidemiological Framework

In addition to the recommendations above, I propose that an intersectional approach (Schulz and Mullings 2005; Bowleg 2012; Rice, Harrison, and Friedman 2019) to epidemiology should be adopted. This approach recognizes and acknowledges that racism is a social determinant of health and it incorporates a Black feminist approach to epidemiology focusing on power and interlocking structural inequality (Bowleg 2021). As Lokot and Avakyan articulate, "An intersectional analysis places power at the center, analyzing not what makes people vulnerable but . . . conceptualizing how power hierarchies and systemic inequalities shape their life experiences" (2020, 3). According to Marcia Inhorn and Lisa Whittle (2001), the conceptual models of epidemiology may reinforce social hierarchies based on gender, race, and class. Lesley Doyal (1995) argues that traditional epidemiological methods have to be turned on their head to understand the complex realities of women's sickness and health. Drawing on Black feminist epistemologies, Inhorn and Whittle propose a feminist epidemiology that privileges four elements: (1) the active engagement of women themselves in the epidemiological knowledge production process; (2) the documentation of women's diverse experiences of illness and health, based on the multiplicity of women's global locations, social and cultural identities, interests, and experiences as both reproductive and nonreproductive human beings; (3) the evaluation of how gender oppression, as well as other interlocking forms of oppression that shape women's daily lives, is itself detrimental to women's health; (4) the connection of women's local lived experiences of health and illness and the various forms of oppression they encounter to larger social, economic, and political forces (2001, 564). The development of Black feminist epidemiological approaches will not only benefit Black women but all women and society as a whole (Douglas 2021). Black women should be involved centrally in developing and implementing epidemiological studies and knowledge production informed by a Black feminist epistemology.

However, Black women scholars in the United Kingdom are to a large extent excluded from research and knowledge production. There are only 35 Black women professors out of 19,285 professors in U.K. universities; this is less than 1 percent of all professors (Advance HE 2019). Black women professors continue to experience racism and microaggressions in their day-to-day experiences in the academy (Rollock 2021). There are limited opportunities for Black women to undertake research and even fewer to lead research. According to UK Research and Innovation (UKRI) data, in relation to research grants, BME researchers were less likely to be awarded research grants as principal investigators than their white colleagues (Baker 2020). Very few BME students are receiving studentships to become academics. In their *Broken Pipeline* report, Williams et al. highlight that over a three-year period, just 1.2 percent of the 19,868 studentships awarded by all UKRI research councils went to Black or Black Mixed students and only 30 of those were from Black Caribbean background (2019, 3).

A Black feminist research tradition is a way of knowing that brings Black women to the center of the analysis and examines Black women's experiences in terms of "race," class, and gender (Mullings 2000). Mirza argues, "Black British feminists reveal *other ways of knowing* that challenge the normative discourse. In our particular world shaped by processes of migration, nationalism, racism, popular culture and the media, black British women, from multiple positions of difference, reveal the distorted ways in which dominant groups construct their assumptions. As black women we see from the sidelines, from our space of unlocation, the unfolding project of domination"

(1997, 5). Black feminist approaches to knowledge production value the lived experience of Black women, recognizing multiple forms of oppression. Developed by Black feminists, intersectionality-informed approaches try to address the complexity of social life by recognizing that individuals simultaneously occupy multiple social locations. A Black feminist epidemiology is concerned with recognizing and documenting multiple, interlocking, and simultaneous forms of oppression in relation to gender, race, class, and nation that women experience.

In collecting epidemiological information, data must be disaggregated in terms of gender and ethnicity. So often it is not, and we do not know how women from particular ethnic groups are experiencing specific health issues such as COVID-19. Epidemiological methodologies and approaches should be developed to explore how race, class, gender, disability, sexuality, sexual orientation, ethnicity, nationality, and citizenship interlock, and that focus on power and structural inequality. As well as collecting and analyzing quantitative data, qualitative methodologies should be used to explore the feelings, experiences, and perceptions of Black women. These experiences should be temporal as well as geographical and spatial, examining and documenting the context in which racial inequities in health are perpetuated.

Conclusion

While we do not have the testimonies of Black women in relation to the 1918–19 influenza pandemic, from the experiences of Nella Larsen it appears there are unequivocal similarities between the experiences of Black women nurses in the early twentieth-century flu pandemic in the United States and those of Black women nurses in the United Kingdom during the COVID-19 pandemic over one hundred years later. In both cases, structural racism, sexism, and discrimination in health services put Black women at greater risk of infection. At the outset of both pandemics, public health doctors jumped first to biological and genetic explanations of disparities in hospitalizations and deaths in Black communities, despite widespread public health knowledge about social determinants of health and long-standing and persistent inequalities in health experienced by Black communities. Hopefully, the COVID-19 pandemic has served to demonstrate that discussion of health inequities must incorporate structural racism as a key component of the social determinants of health.

Black women in the United Kingdom are situated in dispersed Diasporic communities and have been unable to see family members in Africa, the United States, and the Caribbean, yet they are hearing of those family members' deaths from COVID-19. The pandemic has caused a huge mental health toll due to fear and anxiety about COVID-19 and grief over family and community members who have died. The loss of so many lives has impacted Black people further by restricting the number of people who are allowed to attend funerals, in communities where funerals are an important part of celebrating and honoring life. Furthermore, the long-term effects of COVID-19 (long COVID), are just emerging and it is being recognized that this may lead to further disability and job losses.

A Black feminist epidemiology is needed not just to research the health and well-being of Black women but to ensure that epidemiology captures the health experiences of all sections of the population and is able to document and analyze intersectional complexities. This means exploring how race, gender, class, and other oppressions intersect while also examining the ways that political, legal, and organizational power enables and perpetuates discrimination in all of its forms. An epidemiological approach that does not invisibilize Black women is essential. We also need to ensure that Black women have access to opportunities to become legitimate producers of knowledge as researchers and professors. In a hundred years, when we face the prospect of another pandemic, Black women should be able to look back and read how Black women in the twenty-first century fared, directly through the voices and experiences of those women. In the future, I hope that Black women will be involved in all levels of epidemiological research and knowledge production and that a Black feminist and intersectional epistemology is firmly embedded in a "new" and more relevant epidemiology.

Bibliography

Advance HE. 2019. *Equality in Higher Education: Staff Statistical Report 2019*. London: Advance HE. https://s3.eu-west-2.amazonaws.com/assets.creode.advancehe-document-manager/documents/advance-he/AdvanceHE_EqHE_Staff_Stats_Report_%202019_1569507134.pdf.

Baker, Simon. 2020. "Ethnic Minority Academics Less Likely to Win UK Research Grants." *Times Higher Education*, June 30, 2020. https://www.timeshighereducation.com/news/ethnic-minority-academics-less-likely-win-uk-research-grants.

Bernard, Jason, director, and David Harewood, presenter. 2021. *Why Is Covid Killing People of Colour?* London: BBC One.

Bourne, Stephen. 2018. *War to Windrush: Black Women in Britain 1939 to 1948*. London: Jacaranda Books.

———. 2019. *Black Poppies: Britain's Black Community and the Great War*. Cheltenham, U.K.: The History Press.

Bowleg, Lisa. 2012. "The Problem with the Phrase *Women and Minorities*: Intersectionality—an Important Theoretical Framework for Public Health." *American Journal of Public Health* 102, no. 7 (July): 1267–73. https://doi.org/10.2105/AJPH.2012.300750.

———. 2021. "Evolving Intersectionality Within Public Heath: From Analysis to Action." *American Journal of Public Health* 111, no. 1 (January): 88–90. https://doi.org/10.2105/AJPH.2020.306031.

Campbell, Lucy. 2021. "Inquest to Be Held into Covid Death of Rail Worker Allegedly Spat at by Customer." *Guardian*, May 7, 2021. https://www.theguardian.com/uk-news/2021/may/07/inquest-to-be-held-into-covid-death-of-rail-worker-allegedly-spat-at-by-customer.

Charity So White. n.d. "Health Inequalities." Accessed June 23, 2022. https://charitysowhite.org/covid19-health-inequalities.

Davis, Thadius. 1994. *Nella Larsen: Novelist of the Harlem Renaissance.* Baton Rouge: Louisiana State University Press.

Douglas, Jenny. 1992. "Black Women's Health Matters." In *Women's Health Matters,* edited by Helen Roberts, 33–46. London: Routledge.

———. 2018. "The Politics of Black Women's Health in the UK—Intersections of 'Race,' Class, and Gender in Policy, Practice, and Research." In *Black Women in Politics: Demanding Citizenship, Challenging Power, and Seeking Justice,* edited by Julia S. Jordan-Zachery and Nikol G. Alexander-Floyd, 49–68. Albany: State University of New York Press.

———. 2019. "Black Women's Activism and Organisation in Public Health—Struggles and Strategies for Better Health and Wellbeing." *Caribbean Review of Gender Studies,* no. 13 (June): 51–68. http://oro.open.ac.uk/59460/.

———. 2021. "Black Women's Health Still Matters." In *More Than Talk: Perspectives of Black and People of Colour (BPOC) Working in Sexual and Reproductive Health (SRH) in the United Kingdom (UK),* edited by Rianna Raymond-Williams and Lama El Khamy, 32–45. Self-published, Amazon Digital Services. Kindle.

———. 2022. "Black Women and Public Health in the UK." In *Black Women and Public Health: Strategies to Name, Locate, and Change Systems of Power,* edited by Stephanie Y. Evans, Sarita K. Davis, Leslie R. Hinkson, and Deanna J. Wathington, 181–94. Albany: State University of New York Press.

Doyal, Lesley. 1995. *What Makes Women Sick: Gender and the Political Economy of Health.* London: Macmillan.

Ford, Megan. 2020. "Exclusive: BME Nurses 'Feel Targeted' to Work on Covid-19 Wards." *Nursing Times,* April 17, 2020. https://www.nursingtimes.net/news /coronavirus/exclusive-bme-nurses-feel-targeted-to-work-on-covid-19 -wards-17-04-2020/.

Fryer, Peter. 2018. *Staying Power: The History of Black People in Britain.* London: Pluto Press.

Gamble, Vanessa N. 2010. "'There Wasn't a Lot of Comforts in Those Days': African Americans, Public Health, and the 1918 Influenza Epidemic." *Public Health Reports (Washington, D.C.: 1974)* 125, supplement 3: 114–22. https:// doi.org/10.1177/00333549101250S314.

Gentleman, Amelia. 2020. *The Windrush Betrayal: Exposing the Hostile Environment.* London: Guardian Faber Publishing.

Godlee, Fiona. 2021. "How Do We Tackle Racism and Inequality?" *British Medical Journal* 373 (April): n1035. https://doi.org/10.1136/bmj.n1035.

Gopal, Dipesh, and Mala Rao. 2021. "Playing Hide and Seek with Structural Racism." *British Medical Journal* 373 (April): n988. https://doi.org/10.1136/bmj.n988.

Green, Jeffrey. 1998. *Black Edwardians: Black People in Britain 1901–1914*. London: Routledge.

Hine, Darlene Clark. 1989. *Black Women in White: Racial Conflict and Cooperation in the Nursing Profession, 1890–1950*. Bloomington: Indiana University Press.

Hutchinson, George. 2006. *In Search of Nella Larsen: A Biography of the Color Line*. Cambridge, MA: Harvard University Press.

Independent SAGE. 2020. *Disparities in the Impact of Covid-19 in Black and Minority Ethnic Populations: Review and Recommendations*. The Independent SAGE Report 6, July 6, 2020. https://www.independentsage.org/wp-content/uploads/2020/09/Independent-SAGE-BME-Report_02July_FINAL.pdf.

Inhorn, Marcia, and Lisa Whittle. 2001. "Feminism Meets the 'New' Epidemiologies: Toward an Appraisal of Antifeminist Biases in Epidemiological Research on Women's Health." *Social Science and Medicine* 53, no. 5 (September) 553–67. https://doi.org/10.1016/S0277-9536(00)00360-9.

ITV News. 2022. "Belly Mujinga: Inquest Won't Consider 'Covid Spit Attack' on Railway Worker Before Her Death." May 27, 2022. https://www.itv.com/news/london/2022-05-27/belly-mujingas-death-inquest-wont-consider-covid-spit-attack.

Jones, Marian Moser, and Matilda Saines. 2019. "The Eighteen of 1918–19: Black Nurses and the Great Flu Pandemic in the United States." *America Journal of Public Health* 109, no. 6 (June): 877–84. https://doi.org/10.2105/AJPH.2019.305003.

Knight, Marian, Kathryn Bunch, Derek Tuffnell, Hemali Jayakody, Judy Shakespeare, Rohit Kotnis, Sara Kenyon, and Jennifer J. Kurinczuk, eds, on behalf of MBRRACE-UK. 2018. *Saving Lives, Improving Mothers' Care: Lessons Learned to Inform Maternity Care from the UK and Ireland Confidential Enquiries into Maternal Deaths and Morbidity 2014–16*. Oxford, U.K.: National Perinatal Epidemiology Unit, University of Oxford.

Larsen, Nella. 1928. *Quicksand*. New York: Alfred A. Knopf.

———. 1929. *Passing*. New York: Alfred A. Knopf.

Lokot, Michelle, and Yeva Avakyan. 2020. "Intersectionality as a Lens to the COVID-19 Pandemic: Implications for Sexual and Reproductive Health in Development and Humanitarian Contexts." *Sex and Reproductive Health Matters* 28, no. 1: e1764748. https://doi.org/10.1080/26410397.2020.1764748.

McKee, M. 2017. "Grenfell Tower Fire: Why We Cannot Ignore the Political Determinants of Health." *British Medical Journal* 357 (June): j2966. https:// doi.org/10.1136/bmj.j2966.

Mirza, Heidi. 1997. *Black British Feminism: A Reader.* London: Routledge.

Mullings, Leith. 2000. "African-American Women Making Themselves: Notes on the Role of Black Feminist Research." *Souls: A Critical Journal of Black Politics, Culture, and Society* 2, no. 4: 18–29. https://doi.org/10.1080/109999 40009362233.

Okland, Helene, and Svenn-Erik Mamelund. 2019. "Race and 1918 Influenza Pandemic in the United States: A Review of the Literature." *International Journal of Environmental Research and Public Health* 16, no. 4 (July): 2487– 504. https://doi.org/10.3390/ijerph16142487.

ONS (Office for National Statistics). 2020. *Coronavirus (COVID-19) Related Deaths by Ethnic Group, England and Wales: 2 March 2020 to 10 April 2020.* London: ONS, May 7, 2020. https://www.ons.gov.uk/peoplepopulationand community/birthsdeathsandmarriages/deaths/articles/coronavirusrelated deathsbyethnicgroupenglandandwales/2march2020to10april2020.

PHE (Public Health England). 2020a. *Disparities in the Risk and Outcomes of COVID-19.* London: PHE, June 2020. https://assets.publishing.service .gov.uk/government/uploads/system/uploads/attachment_data/file/908 434/Disparities_in_the_risk_and_outcomes_of_COVID_August_2020 _update.pdf.

———. 2020b. *Beyond the Data: Understanding the Impact of COVID-19 on BAME Groups.* London: PHE, June 2020. https://assets.publishing.service .gov.uk/government/uploads/system/uploads/attachment_data/file/892376 /COVID_stakeholder_engagement_synthesis_beyond_the_data.pdf.

Rice, Carla, Elisabeth Harrison, and May Friedman. 2019. "Doing Justice to Intersectionality in Research." *Cultural Studies ↔ Critical Methodologies* 19, no. 6: 409–20. https://doi.org/10.1177/1532708619829779.

Rollock, Nicola. 2021. "'I Would Have Become Wallpaper Had Racism Had Its Way': Black Female Professors, Racial Battle Fatigue, and Strategies for Surviving Higher Education." *Peabody Journal of Education* 96, no. 2 (May): 206–17. https://doi.org/10.1080/0161956X.2021.1905361.

Schulz, Amy, and Leith Mullings. 2005. *Gender, Race, Class and Health: Intersectional Approaches.* New York: Jossey-Bass.

Slater, Ross, and Nick Fagge. 2020. "Eight-Month Pregnant Nurse Mary, Who Died of Coronavirus but Whose Baby Was Saved, Lost Her Father 'to Virus'

Just Two Weeks Ago." *Daily Mail*, April 16, 2020. https://www.dailymail.co
.uk/news/article-8226319/Pregnant-nurse-28-died-coronavirus-baby-saved
-lost-father-Covid-19.html.

Stafford, Mai, Usha Boolaky, Tim Elwell-Sutton, Miqdad Asaria, and James
Nazroo. 2020. *How to Interpret Research on Ethnicity and COVID-19 Risk
and Outcomes: Five Key Questions*. London: Health Foundation, August 27,
2020. https://www.health.org.uk/publications/long-reads/how-to-interpret
-research-on-ethnicity-and-covid-19-risk-and-outcomes-five.

Williams, Paulette, Sukhi Bath, Jason Arday, and Chantelle Lewis. 2019. *The
Broken Pipeline: Barriers to Black PhD Students Accessing Research Council Funding*. London: Leading Routes. https://leadingroutes.org/mdocs
-posts/the-broken-pipeline-barriers-to-black-students-accessing-research
-council-funding.

CHAPTER 4

Wanawake Wavumilivu

Tanzanian Women's Voices of Survivance

Amber Walker and Rhonda M. Gonzales

Introduction

Wanawake wavumilivu translates from Kiswahili into English as "women who persevere" or "women who endure." The voices that amplify this essay tell a story of how Tanzanian women embody the ideals of survivance, which we choose to define as survival through resistance. In this case, Tanzanian women were resisting government denial of COVID-19 by taking measures that ensure the safety of their own homes and communities, resisting the indecisiveness of the Centers for Disease Control and Prevention (CDC) and the World Health Organization (WHO) through shared knowledge of traditional and ancestral medicine, and resisting through surviving under a colonial structure that predicted a grave loss of life on the African continent (Nordling 2020). The act of not being passive recipients of colonialism but rather maneuvering through the tools of colonialism to ensure survival is a pillar of survivance.

Survivance is often theorized through conversations of Native American existence, storytelling, and maintaining connections to history, while curtailing the narrative that Indigenous communities were exterminated by the evils of colonialism. Survivance, as it has been conceptualized, embodies resistance in that it centers the experiences of communities and their inherent need to overcome adversities imposed through colonialism, as a way of sustaining histories, cultures, and traditions, thus reverting the community to its autochthonous state. Writer Gerald Vizenor (2009) explains in *Native Liberty: Natural Reason and Cultural Survivance* that survivance upholds communal responsibility and being presently active in maintaining community livelihood; unlike survival, which is based on minimally existing in spite of circumstances, survivance acknowledges the dynamic and power in Indigenous storytelling and the work people do to carry those stories forward.

Survivance in this context would be best supported through literature by Tanzanian women theorizing their own historical experiences, but the absence of such literature in academia is the reason for this essay's pertinence. To fill this gap, we are extending the conversation of survivance to the context of Tanzanian women and focusing on ways they resist dominant authority and expectations in society. Specifically, we explore how Black Tanzanian women displayed survivance in their daily lives during the COVID-19 pandemic by resisting the paternal nature of a government that withheld vital information about the pandemic and thus hindered the ability of Tanzanians to learn about COVID-19 protocols and choose whether or not to follow them. Instead, President John Magufuli downplayed the global impact and seriousness of coronavirus. Magufuli's decision to hide Tanzania's COVID-19 statistics rejected the narrative that Tanzania would suffer.

The death-driven narrative laid out by the West failed to materialize and the country avoided extreme infection rates because Tanzanians committed to each other, embraced traditional medicines, and maintained distance from tourists. This essay expounds on the ways that women in the community have been leading such efforts. The hindrances encountered by the women featured in this essay, and the decisions they made in resistance, serve as a lens through which we can view survivance in Tanzania. Some of the women we interviewed expressed their disappointment with a lack of government intervention but also shared the precautions they took in order to protect their families. Eila, who will be introduced shortly, shared her frustration with the government:

> It's just, I wish the government would have been more open despite just reporting the numbers. Let the people decide whether they want to stay inside or go out, but at least if they know that this is how serious it is, or this is how it's trending, we're getting less cases or getting more. Kind of trust them with that information to make their own decisions and make them make smart decisions. But to lie about that.

Eila's opinion is representative of how Magufuli's paternalism was felt among the community. The Tanzanian government's response to the COVID-19 crisis is inextricably linked to its ongoing public health challenges. Magufuli held a PhD in chemistry and thus was educated in the importance of science-informed decision-making. Yet his approach to the expected pandemic largely centered on minimizing COVID-19's potential threat. Magufuli defended his position, saying he used a PCR test to swab samples from a papaya, a quail, and a goat, labeled them with human names, sent them into the lab for COVID testing, and because some returned COVID-positive results, he claimed that labs could not be trusted (*The Citizen* 2020b). In early June 2020, Magufuli doubled down further, declaring that Tanzania was free of coronavirus because God responded through prayer. He said, "I want to thank Tanzanians of all faiths. We have been praying and fasting for God to save us from the pandemic that has afflicted our country and the world. God has answered us. The coronavirus disease has been eliminated by God" (BBC News 2020). Tanzania had not reported COVID-19 infection numbers to the CDC since April 29, 2020; the U.S. Embassy reports the World Health Organization began receiving "limited aggregated weekly numbers" from the Tanzanian government September 2021 (U.S. Embassy Dar es Salaam

2021). In March 2021, John Magufuli, who was not seen in public for the two weeks prior, was announced dead by the succeeding president, Samia Suluhu Hassan. Following Hassan's inauguration as the first woman president of Tanzania, she announced stricter measures to fight further COVID-19 outbreaks and aid in Tanzania's return to global society (Sippy 2021). President Hassan's actions replicate those of the responsibilities taken on by women in Tanzanian society.

This display of reversing Magufuli's misjudgment, which protects society as a whole, can be viewed through gendered discussions of the ways that women, even those in power, handle crisis situations in comparison to men. This essay paints a picture of survivance in Tanzania through the conversation of women's resistance, making it salient for us to gender survivance and proclaim that Black women in Tanzania are cornerstones of their communities; their methods of resistance embody the theory of survivance. Survivance is shown through Black women who experience moments of tragedy yet create spaces and opportunities, often anchored in historical, local ways of knowing that are adapted to contemporary contexts so that they might thrive in the face of adversity. In this essay, we analyze a series of interviews that reveal how Black women in Tanzania have navigated a global pandemic and illustrate how they exhibit survivance. Capturing the voices of Black women in Tanzania during this historical moment provides observances missed during the flu pandemic a century ago and viewing them through the lens of survivance pushes us to examine the ways in which women in Africa have been historically discussed.

The COVID-19 pandemic led to global shutdowns, emerging mental health crises, and apprehension about the future, but these women show us how they maintained agency and resilience to push through by creating ways to cope, leaning on their talents, skills, and faith, and maintaining agency through resistance. This work steps away from positioning Black women as victims under the hands of government decisions and patriarchy during the pandemic and proclaims that, in spite of these uncontrollable circumstances, the women protected their vested interests, which maintained community. This approach does not negate Black women's historical and present experiences of marginalization or subjugation but rather takes the position that though a global pandemic amplified these experiences, women retained and wielded agency through methods of resistance and survivance.

Voice

Due to shutdowns, we recruited for the interviews virtually and by word of mouth. We requested Black women we know in Tanzania, or who are from Tanzania, to interview and to ask their friends who identify as Black Tanzanian women if they would be interested in sharing their stories. Prior to organizing times to interview, we successfully completed Institutional Review Board (IRB) training and approvals. Initial screening questions asked about how women identified to ensure each woman fit the description of what was required for this essay, and then substantive questions asked details about their experiences during the pandemic (see appendix A at the end of this chapter for questions).

Profiles of each woman are provided here with the understanding that such knowledge is essential to their experiences and to honor their voices, ways of knowing, and worldviews.[1] Two of the nine women interviewed, Mya and Ezette, were not born in Tanzania, but they had lived in the country for a minimum of three years. Mya was born and raised in the United States and has lived in a few countries on the African continent. She has lived on Zanzibar Island for three years, where she was working as a teacher; she had to quit her job at the beginning of the pandemic due to a lack of funding to purchase internet cards that would permit her to teach virtually. During this time, Mya suffered from what doctors presumed was COVID-19, but testing revealed she had actually contracted E. coli. Following her illness, she tutored a former student for two months, earning sixty dollars per week. Ezette was born in Liberia but grew up in the United States from the age of five. She lives in Zanzibar with her child, where she leads a private school. Prior to the pandemic, she was planning to return to the United States and visit her parents, and voiced, during the interview, that her child constantly questioned when they would be able to visit his grandmother.

The remaining seven women are Tanzanian natives, but their experiences and travels vary, providing us with a spectrum of understanding about the ways Tanzanian Black women are living through the pandemic. Eila was born in northern Tanzania but lived with family in the United States and East Africa throughout her childhood. She currently lives in Dar es Salaam, Tanzania's largest metropolitan city, where she works as an administrative assistant for an international entity. During the pandemic, she has been the sole provider for her mother and four younger siblings. Tamu was born and raised in Tanzania but when we spoke with her, she had been living in North America for two years to pursue her education. She has three children; her youngest child lives with Tamu's husband in Tanzania. Lilith is a script writer from Dar es Salaam, who lives with her one child and elderly parents. She was unable to make money through scriptwriting, so she started a small business selling ice cream to the neighborhood children. At the time of her interview, she shared that her parents were earning some income from the homes they rented to people. Salma is from the island of Pemba, Tanzania's smaller archipelago, but she lives in Zanzibar where she is a teacher. During the pandemic, she earned income by transitioning to online teaching. She cares for her four children alone, in addition to caring for her sister's three children. Hava is Zanzibari, meaning she was born on the island, and as a student, she depends on her mother for financial support, but her mother has been unable to conduct her trade business during the pandemic. Fatima is a journalism student from Dar es Salaam. Prior to the pandemic, she earned money by producing YouTube videos and completing broadcast journalism jobs. Once the pandemic began, she finished any work virtually, but very soon after that, when Tanzanians returned to their normal lives, she was not allowed by her brother to continue the work she previously did and had to stay home, thus not earning any income. She and her sister have been staying in their brother's home to ensure their safety, and he has been providing for their essentials. She shared her discomfort with asking her brother for money to buy feminine products. Lastly, Takama is Zanzibari and lives with her one-year-old child. During the pandemic, she has continued working as a teacher's assistant, earning the equivalent of one hundred dollars per month. The backgrounds of each woman aid in framing their perspectives.[2] The way these stories are told, experiences of the women, and expectations amid a global pandemic are shaped by their status in Tanzanian society. They have attained formal education, and four of the nine have parents who are university educated, and three of those four have parents and siblings who are medical professionals.

Gendering Survivance

In the context of Tanzanian society, women's preeminent role as community leaders, mothers, and caregivers is critical to the growth of societal structures. Historically, Western-framed conversations regarding the position of African women have placed them in presumed victimhood under the thumb of colonial patriarchy. Professor of African history Christine Saidi analyzes the impact of feminism on the Western perception of women in African societies, saying that second-wave feminism has reinforced the "myth of the universal oppression of women" (2010, 11). This myth asserts that all women worldwide experience oppression in the same manner, and if women in the so-called developed world with civilized societies suffer oppression, then women in subaltern societies must suffer substantially more oppression and are in need of saving.

This perspective ignores the incomparable role African women play in maintaining the livelihoods of their communities, specifically the ways they obtain necessities like food, water, and money to survive. Historically, they have preserved their communities through paid and unpaid labor, household care, farming, business ownership, etc. This essay centers the experiences of Black women. Understanding the ways intersectional identities impact Black women globally, it felt imperative to inquire about their experiences during the pandemic in comparison to men and non-Black women in their communities. When asked if they noticed differences between the lives of men and women during the pandemic, the women shared key differences in the ways Tanzanian men navigated finding jobs in a market that had become tighter for women than for men, and noted men's freedom to not shelter in place due to patriarchal double standards. When asked about differences between Black Tanzanian women and non-Black women, the consistent response reflected an absence of non-Black women within the communities. Lilith answered, for example, "I did not see, because there are no white people where I live." This shows a separation of race and gender in colonial order; European women being oppressed as European women does not equate to the marginalization, inferiorization, and exploitation of African women whose encounters are based on both Africanness and womanness. A few of the women extended their response to include an interpretation of the way specific Black women were impacted. Eila, for instance, shared knowledge of a woman in her community:

There's this lady who has a little grocery kiosk right next to my house. She's a single mom, but she had to [work], she got diabetes, she's underweight. She kept coming to work every morning setting up her little shop, and didn't have masks on, I think that she wasn't the only woman that had to do that. A lot of women work in the market who have to go daily to get food for their children. We have a lot of single women here, single mothers. That was something that they couldn't afford— not to go to work.

This narrative, through the lens of survivance, can be seen as the sedulous continuation of a habit rather than a struggle. The necessity of a Tanzanian woman to keep her grocery in operation not only to sustain herself and family but to also feed the community during a time of insecurity around the world shows survivance. However, Eila's interpretation showcases a capitalist contradiction that forces one to choose between health and livelihood, between getting coronavirus by working or being unable to sustain a livelihood by not working.

This is inextricably linked to survivance, as our introduction defines it, survival through resistance. This does not negate the oppressiveness of patriarchy but sets a stance that African women are not passive victims in society. Gendered divisions that hamper African women's contributions impact the whole of society, but efforts of the women to survive show their inherent value in societal structures, including the economy (Clark 2019). In "The State of Women in Tanzania," American scholar, feminist, and gender activist Marjorie Mbilinyi writes that the oppressive nature of men has been integrated into Tanzanian society over time, stating, "Male resistance against all efforts in the direction of 'women's emancipation' is outspoken, influential and represents the attitudes of the majority of Tanzanian men" (1972, 372). This generalized argument reveals the Western position of feminism taken by Mbilinyi and ignores the historical knowledge that women play a major role in the distribution of authority, power, and material wealth of their lineages. Mbilinyi follows with the statement that "women have been taught to be passive in the face of opposition. They also tend to be isolated from one another by class, tribal, and marital divisions. They need to develop a consciousness of their own historical position and a will for unified action as well as organization" (372). The actions and stories of each woman we interviewed contest the passiveness Mbilinyi speaks of, through their demonstration of survivance through resistance, the use of traditional medicine, and coping mechanisms.

Survivance Is Agency Through Resistance

This section explores the theory of survivance through Tanzanian women's resistance of false narratives that endanger their lives during a global pandemic. The women featured in this section share stories of how they reacted to learning about the coronavirus outbreak, the government's denial of COVID-19, precautions they took to protect their families, and their unwillingness to accept subpar directives from the government.

After gathering demographic information, we asked the women about the changes in their daily lives, how they responded to hearing about COVID-19, and how their lives were impacted. Salma, when asked whether her normal activities changed after learning about coronavirus, explained, "When I heard COVID was spreading from country to country, I thought [about] what would happen because Tanzania is poor, but we prayed a lot and Allah accepted our prayers and we are all right." Although Salma did not refute the government's stance that coronavirus was not in Tanzania due to God removing it, she took actions to protect herself, thus claiming agency for her and her family's own well-being in the face of government messaging. Salma exhibits survivance in her reflection about changes she experienced with the onset of COVID and the government response. When asked about her feeling regarding the government's denial she replied,

There are things you need to think about by yourself and don't expect leaders or the government to tell you everything to do. Once I heard about this coronavirus, I started to look [at] how I can protect myself and my family. And even my other brothers and sisters—they were doing the same, so we communicate what to do to be safe, so we say don't visit each other, let's use email or WhatsApp, but let's stop visiting each other until this over.

Hava responded similarly yet was explicit in her doubt of the government while also offering possible rationale for their approach, saying, "I don't know if there are patients the government is hiding. I don't think so. I don't know. Our government is trying to keep us calm, but still there is not any sign of anything showing that corona is here." While Hava offered rationale for the government's behavior, she does acknowledge that places like Zanzibar, Tanzania's archipelago, is small enough to avoid unrestrained outbreaks of coronavirus, so whether the government is lying is contestable, as there is no evidence to prove otherwise. Her observations were also shared by Ezette, who observed the size of the island and lack of travel as factors that limited the spread of COVID.

Each woman held unique, sometimes doubtful, perspectives of the government, yet some expressed a sense of gratitude that Tanzania's COVID situation was not dire. Mya, who did not shelter in place, explained that in her conversations with Zanzibaris, she repeatedly heard that coronavirus was just another disease. She said, "It was never a big deal here. People say we have malaria, cholera, another disease isn't gonna make a difference, we're still going to survive. We are used to dealing with these situations." This perspective brings into question whether the government's reaction was based on the reality that Tanzania has a long epidemiological history dealing with epidemics like HIV, malaria, and cholera, and a long history of dealing with the ramifications of Western intervention; these histories might cause the government to reject interactions with the United States and European nations as a way of community protection (Makoni 2021).

Comparatively, African countries, altogether, fared much better than the Americas, Europe, and South Asia in COVID-19 cases; community health care, quick action, and public support for safety measures are among the reasons identified by researchers (Soy 2020).

Eila, who lives in Dar es Salaam, revealed that her family members who are nurses kept the family updated about the state of COVID-19 in Tanzania but did so quietly for fear of government retaliation. Eila's fears of coronavirus spreading through communities of deniers, conspiracy theorists, and government supporters became reality when she began showing symptoms of COVID-19. Working in an international environment, her boss was supportive in sending her home until she recovered. In Eila's interview, there were a few follow-up questions about her family being health-care workers, how she felt regarding hearing these government contradictions, and how she dealt with the reality of possibly receiving a false negative on the COVID-19 test.

She shared, "Recently, they [Tanzanian government] said this big second wave of COVID [is coming] and [they] are getting more positives. Of course, we're not allowed to say that." Acknowledging the limit placed on her speech by government officials, then planning around those limits, Eila demonstrated her refusal to simply spectate while being directly impacted by the virus. She continued, "You know, sometimes [I heard] really tough stories about patients who were really sick—elderly, especially, were really sick—and they couldn't be with their family members, because they had to be in quarantine."

Explaining how she dealt with this reality, she said, "It really sucks, because a family member of mine is working in an environment that is unsafe. And [the government is] here telling me that there are no cases, no new cases, yet any day, one of my family members could be the newest case." Her words outrightly rejected the government's interference with individual autonomy.

Answering a question about her ability to protect herself in an environment that largely denies COVID-19's existence, she shared,

At work we have to wear masks. So, we do that. Actually, funny enough. Last Thursday, last week, I lost my sense of taste and smell. And I told my boss and I had to go get tested and I had to quarantine. It's awkward because my family lives with me. So there's this extra room of sorts. I had to move out some things, and kind of holed myself [up] in there.

She continued to share about the testing experience in Dar es Salaam:

I got tested at the Aga Khan hospital, which is an okay hospital and it's a private hospital. I walked in and this guy was not wearing a mask while working in that facility for testing. I went with my mask on, and I did not want to get anyone sick, in case I was. So I gave this guy my paper. Then they called me in, and I had to line up, no social distancing. No social distancing, no physical distancing, but I kind of prepared myself mentally. It's gonna suck. It's going to be getting my brain picked. So they did that thing. They told me when my results would be ready and how I could get them. And I walked out and came back two days later to get my results in a crowded room, not room but outdoor-ish, but no physical distance. The people on the other side of the counter were not wearing masks. Everyone was kind of huddled next to the little windows trying to get their receipts in so they could get the results. It was strange, because it was a big question of what if I tested positive and, you know, I'm not wearing gloves, but you're not [either]. We're exchanging so many things. I was disappointed at the lack of precaution that they were taking. But if that's a private institution, I can imagine what it's like in public hospitals.

I asked what her other symptoms were, and she shared,

Lack of taste and smell and I didn't have the flu. I don't. When I told my boss, he probably thought that it's a false negative. And a little bit of me suspects that it was but it's also strange that I didn't have any other symptoms. I didn't have a fever. No fatigue—that's out of the ordinary. But I've never lost a sense of taste or smell in that way. It's usually the flu and I have a stuffy nose. It was about a week and two days, and then slowly my sense of taste started coming back. And I have to give my mother thanks here because when I was holed up in that room, she'd always bring me some lemon ginger, herbal mixes of all sorts that matured on a bowl of ginger, like "better finish that." But yeah, she really worked hard to give me my sense of taste and smell back. And now actually [my sense of smell is] not really fully back, but my sense of taste is back. I'm hoping that it was a false negative and that I didn't pass it on to any of my family members. And I really hope it doesn't happen to anyone else. No. I could have been lucky that I had my own symptoms if I actually had it. But I know how bad it can get in some ways.

Eila's story exemplifies survivance not only in her commitment to implicate Tanzanian leadership for denying the impact of COVID-19 on the community but identifying the pattern of problems created by the government's perceived negligence. She also demonstrated survivance by advocating for herself and family, highlighting the caring nature of her mother, and thanking her mother for the work she put into ensuring Eila's recovery. These traits exist within many Tanzanian women who hold value in nurturing the communities they build.

Other difficulties the women featured in this essay overcame included gaining access to common necessities like menstrual pads. Menstrual pads are an expensive product in Tanzania, and access is a problem for young women globally. Pads can be found in shops, but it is more common for women to wear the traditional cloth as protection. Women and girls in Tanzania often use a *kanga* because the price of menstrual pads is so high. The East African *kanga* is a thin, colorful cotton cloth often printed with quotes and witty Kiswahili sayings, and has historically been used as an object of versatility. *Kangas* are used as hijabs (Muslim women's headscarves), table coverings, bath towels, floor mats, clothing, menstrual protection, and in other myriad ways. The women interviewed for this essay revealed that during this pandemic, there was a need to return to the use of a *kanga* during menstruation due to lack of money or limited product. Hava shared her experience with needing to return to it. "We use *kangas* to help us during those times, so it was kind of difficult. We used to use pads, but now we don't have money, we [can't] go out, so we use *kangas*." Returning to the use of *kangas* to replace pads, Hava shared, "felt weird, crazy. . . . It's not comfortable the way it is with a pad but still you don't have any other way and our elders will say it's okay we use *kangas*." Of the nine women we interviewed, four returned to using cloth due to lack of access to pads.

Similar to a *kanga*, a *vitambaa* is another type of cloth. Fatima detailed an experience she had with needing to use *vitambaa*, as well the experiences of women around her.

There were some things I wasn't able to ask of my brother because his wife wasn't there . . . some things I couldn't tell him because he's a man and sometimes I felt like we were being a burden to him. Like pads, sometimes he brings them home but when they are finished, I wasn't able to ask [for more]. I feel like I'm being a burden so I will use other means like *vitambaa*. We have to have many pieces. You have to make sure you wash them, iron them; it was [more] difficult than using a pad. I created some pieces for me and my little sister, but the housemaid was wearing like three or four pants to stop the blood from falling out.

The commodification of women's menstrual cycles results in decreased accessibility based on class. Menstrual pads are sold in most shops and cost an average of 3,000 Tanzanian shillings (TSH) for a pack of eight; that is an average of $1.50 USD. From the Western lens, $1.50 USD for pads seems relatively low priced, but eight pads are not enough for the average menstrual cycle, which can last seven to eight days, because the pad needs to be changed more than once a day. Therefore, women would need to purchase two or three packs of pads to securely, and hygienically, care for their periods, making the true price 9,000 TSH ($4.50 USD) per menstrual cycle. A single *kanga* or *vitambaa* can average between 4,000 TSH ($2 USD) and 40,000 TSH ($20 USD) depending on the size. When using cloth, women cut it into pieces, as Fatima shares above, and use it to line their panties. The use of cloth can lead to infection if there is a lack of water to clean it. Women in Tanzania earn less than men, and the Tanzania National Bureau of Labor Statistics reported in 2018 that women made an average of $38 per month, and those who work domestic labor as household maids in rural areas could earn as little as $13 per month. Tanzania's average minimum wage for professional jobs, inclusive of men and women, is $100 per month. Therefore, menstrual necessities cost women more than what they can afford. Women should not have to pay for menstrual care. What Fatima's account reveals is that the cost of menstrual care, even for traditional, more affordable methods, is not accessible to all (Kottasová 2018).

She continued to explain an incident where a neighbor came to her brother's house seeking water, possibly needing it due to her menstruation, but, as the women prepared to help her, her brother refused to give the neighbor water due to fear of catching COVID-19. Fatima's position in her brother's home prevented her from helping another, but her insistence and protesting, though unsuccessful, truly reveals the impact of community among women in Tanzania.

One day this neighbor came and knocked at our gate. She wanted water, we tried to let her in but when bro came and actually saw us fetch the water, he was so angry, like why are you doing this there's COVID, people are dying, and we're like, bro, COVID will end and she is your neighbor and he said no you're not allowed to let anyone in and you're not allowed to go out—even if anything happens, you're not allowed to go out. She needed water but we couldn't help her because bro said we can't take the risk; we have small children here.

Fatima's sensitivity to the ways that access to water directly impacts women and their ability to maintain hygiene, protect themselves from disease, and provide for their children likely influenced her defense of the neighbor. Following up about the neighbor's reaction to her brother refusing water, she indicated the neighbor tried to convince him to "give her even one bucket, but he said, you can go somewhere else." Because she was clearly emphatic about helping the neighbor, I asked how this incident may have impacted her. She shared,

It did really affect me, because we women need water and I think what if I was in her place and I needed that water. Maybe I'm on my period and I need water to clean myself, but you face a situation where you can't get even one bucket of water and we couldn't make my brother understand she needs the water, so I felt bad about that. Women are the ones that faced the very challenging moment during the pandemic.

More knowledgeable and empathetic to the ways women are impacted by a lack of resources than her brother, Fatima's account shows us the struggles Tanzanian women face during the pandemic: they have extremely limited access to jobs, food, hygiene products, and water, while still being expected to care for children, families, and communities.

Survivance Is Agency Through Traditional Medicine

Tanzanian women's use of natural or traditional medicines is one demonstration of survivance during the coronavirus outbreak. Communities embrace the use of natural medicines and actively use plants often to heal ailments. Embracing those traditions during a time of informational insecurity created soundness and community reliability with this shared knowledge. According to the WHO, "Traditional medicine is the sum total of all knowledge and practices, whether explicable, or not, used in diagnosis, prevention, and elimination of physical, mental, or social imbalance and relying exclusively on practical experience handed down from generation to generation whether verbally or in writing" (2019). Class distinctions determine historical claims to drug discovery, creating a knowledge hierarchy where scientific discovery is desired over traditional medicine. Scientific historian Abena Osseo-Asare refers to this as "scientific appropriation" (2014, 17). Where this process focuses on written data collection for testing plants, traditional medicine is knowledge passed down through generations via oral tradition. In African societies, oral tradition as a way of keeping, passing, and maintaining knowledge does not need to be written. Africanists Rhonda Gonzales, Catherine Fourshey, and Christine Saidi explain that the passing down of historical traditions through Bantu languages was not written until the nineteenth century, in what they refer to as the preservation of "old knowledge" (2018, 109). In writing about survivance through the use of tradition and ritual, this essay recognizes the use of traditional medicine to combat and ward off coronavirus, understanding that the choice to use medicinal herbs is upholding survivance. During the interviews, a few women mentioned the use of a process called steaming, where one boils a formula of plants, covers one's head with a blanket or towel, and inhales the vapors.

During the interviews, the women were asked to share any traditions, beliefs, or knowledge they had prior to the coronavirus outbreak that helped them during the pandemic. Their answers demonstrated the relationship between religious beliefs, traditions, and ancestral knowledge. Salma set a strict set of rules for what her household would do, despite government messages.

The country didn't have lockdown, so everyone was walking as nor-mal, [going] to market, but I took my own transport, wearing masks, wearing a niqab. After returning home from buying food, I asked [the] children to not touch anything and to stay outside while I clean and removed clothes; [I] put [Dettol] in a special bowl to wash clothes and body. Drinking ginger tea with lime, preparing different kinds of leaves, boiling them, and covering [your]self—this helps to feel fresh. [Take] tea leaves, lime leaves, *mwarobaini* leaves,[3] then boil until smoke comes and cover [your]self to inhale smoke. Once you finish using it, you feel you are free from something, like something changes in the body; you can use these things for inhaling, drinking, or showering. *Bibis* in the village give you leaves.

Salma's inclination to lean into local village remedies and treatments rooted in inherited knowledge is an example of the enduring lega-cies that medicine and healing perpetuate. These legacies belong to deeply rooted Bantu epistemologies that have been passed between generations of family, specifically from grandmothers to their lineal granddaughters.

Lilith shared her process for steaming, and though the purpose is the same, she used a few different leaves than Salma. She explains,

We steamed ourselves. Steaming was very helpful for me, but other people lost their life because of steaming. They say if you have a certain disease, you shouldn't be steaming yourself, like blood pressure, heart attack, and others. You take some leaves, lemon leaves, you cut some lemons, also some lemongrass, ginger, then you boil the mixture in water and when it is very hot you take a blanket and cover yourself, so you breathe that steam. When I felt heavy, I did that and I felt very good, but for somebody like my dad, [they can] get very sick. I heard some people lost their life. Also, we use seeds of pumpkins. They are very helpful for immunity. [And take] the seeds of avocado and mix with tea. The avocado seed, you take them off and wash them and make as you make groundnuts. The avocado seed, you grind it, dry it in the sun, and then you mix it [with tea].

Takama's response, however, came when asking what gave her hope during the pandemic. She expressed how the use of this traditional steaming is what provided her with hope for the future. It was a reminder that using such traditional remedies during a global pandemic is maintaining agency and intentionality. Takama shared, "After I heard that those people who had corona are okay, I get hope. Also, when the president announced we have to take it like other diseases, I get hope. When I heard we can take local medicine, I had hope." When asked to elaborate on what she meant by "local medicine," Takama said,

We are using some plants and boil them, like three or four types, or five, and then we boil them and those smoke from that boiled medicine and then you cover all your body and then the smoke enters into every part of the body. One day I started to feel like I had the flu and I started to think maybe I have corona and I start to use those Nungu, we call Nungu, those plants. I smoke and the next day I was okay. The flu was gone.

The use of this remedy shows how Tanzanian women use the wisdom granted to them through community consciousness and shared familial knowledge, to survive a global pandemic.

Survivance Is Agency Through Coping

Navigating the celerity of a global pandemic caused an initial reaction of disbelief as the world awaited next steps and direction from health officials worldwide. Although circumstances varied for each woman, they all expressed the feeling of shock when asked whether COVID-19 made them change their daily activities. Tamu shared,

> It surely did. I stopped working, school became virtual, [it] just became haunting to even go out to do grocery shopping. From the point of getting outside my door to going to the supermarket inside, it was daunting. So everything just changed. It felt like, what do you call it? Like the end of the world. It was depressing and scary. The uncertainty was immense and not knowing what's gonna happen, but that's when I learned to basically have faith.

Fatima, whose brother is a doctor, shared a similar feeling of insecurity and dread during the start of the pandemic, saying,

> I was scared when I heard of COVID, thought it was the end, we will never return to school. We sheltered at my brother's house. We were strictly prohibited to go out of the house. We never went out of the house until universities opened. Our brother was telling us, COVID is real, I see it at the hospital, people are dying, it not safe.

Mya's perspective about living in Tanzania during the pandemic was pragmatic. When questioned about living in Tanzania during this global crisis, she informed us, "First I was nervous and scared about not having adequate health care, but that's a risk you take when you are overseas. I feel like this is my home and I don't feel any way about it." The worldview she developed as a result of these events followed the same sentiment.

> Western countries don't know how to handle big emergencies like this, and they were all anticipating there were going to be so many dead in Africa and they're gonna suffer so much, but maybe we are all resilient here. I kind of have hope in Zanzibar. I can survive here. If the world ends, I can learn to fish. I'll be fine. I never felt short of resources or

panicked, because the community looks out for each other, and they have accepted me. I just knew that no matter what, I will be okay. We are all human and will figure it out and survive.

Mya's standpoint really shows the impacts of communal trust and allows us to embrace the ways in which survivance is reflected through that trust. Mya's resistance is in identifying how Western countries engage in individualistic authority, and although born in the West, she embraces Zanzibar as her home, which means also embracing community.

The women described in this essay truly embraced their talents and passions to help them cope with the realities of the pandemic. Ezette, who runs a school, grappled with having to plan for both her students and her child, but as the intensity of the pandemic wore off in Tanzania, she expressed that she felt safer in Zanzibar than she would have in the United States.

I did feel confident in Zanzibar, because when I was like, Okay, I see that they're taking action. Handwashing stations are all over the town, in villages, in the city, in Stone Town. On top of that, there was a [WHO] WhatsApp number that was circulated, you would just send a code to that number, and then it would give you updates based on your region. I was feeling more confident and safer here than [I would have with] what was happening in the States.

The final interview question asked the women what worldview they developed due to this pandemic and how they maintained control. Their responses were filled with compassion. Tamu said,

I feel like there's always these voices. The reason why we become powerless and out of control is because we got these voices telling us like, it's this and you just got to shut down those voices, you have to basically just find ways to shut them down. And I attest that it can be done. It can be done. I have like a thousand voices telling me otherwise. And I managed to shut them down just by urging me to just say, Hey, I need to do something for myself. Nobody else is gonna do it for me. If I don't do it, no one will. So that kept me going.

Ezette, who began to struggle with depression as the pandemic lingered, shared,

> The main thing is to find some kind of purpose, however big, however small. Because if you think that you're not connected to the world, or what you're doing has no impact on anybody else or anything, then it's almost like you're isolating yourself from everything, right? For me, it was just knowing that my actions, like I'm staying at home, and even though I can't see the other people at least I felt some kind of solace. And that, yeah, we're all in this together. My purpose is I have to make sure that I'm taking care of myself, so that I can take care of my child. So, then my purpose became greater than just taking care of myself, taking care of my son. I still want to be a citizen of the world. Just start with something small that you care about, or something within you that you still want to see happen.

Ezette took her own advice, and by the end of the pandemic, she had published a storybook about her and her son's experience living in Tanzania during a global crisis. Her way of adapting through creativity, and producing a tangible outcome, is a guide through which we can view ways that Black women emanate survivance through coping during the coronavirus pandemic.

Conclusion

Conversations that center survivance often reflect the nature in which Indigenous people have resisted systems of oppression on their land.

This essay brings Africa into that conversation through Black women's stories of pushing back at systems of authority that do not account for their welfare during a global pandemic. It navigates a conversation that seeks to answer what survivance is in the Tanzanian context and how Black women are the embodiment of that survivance—survival through an intentional resistance that protects communal interests. This essay shows how Tanzanian women exhibit the theory of survivance through numerous ways: the women's conscious decisions to take precautions to protect their families from coronavirus by acknowledging that the government is not entirely truthful in their discussion of COVID statistics; Fatima's struggle to convince her brother to share water with a neighbor; the government's stance on COVID-19 prompting the women to use traditional medicine, a knowledge historically passed through grandmothers; Eila caring for her family, and in turn having her mom care for her while she recovered from COVID-19. These women resisted in reticence, ensuring the overall protection of their families and communities. The interviews of each woman show how they were impacted by coronavirus in numerous ways—whether losing their jobs, getting ill, losing family members, suffering with loneliness and mental health, or being forced to stay away from their children—but the power and control held by each woman during times of challenges and revelations shows how survivance is based on community, resistance, and perseverance.

Appendix A: Interview Questions and Script

Hello. Thank you for your willingness to participate in this oral history project on COVID-19 and Tanzanian women's experiences.

This oral history project wishes to hear the stories of Black women who have lived in Tanzania and their experiences during the coronavirus outbreak. Thank you for allowing us to hear your story. At the beginning of the interview, I will ask your name and permission to record the interview. I remind you that your name and other identifiers will not be used in any publication.

1. Do you give me permission to record this interview with the understanding that no identifying information will be used in any publication?
2. Please state your name.
3. What is your age?
4. Do you identify as a woman?
5. What is your profession?
6. What languages do you speak?
7. Were you born in Tanzania?
8. Have you ever lived in Tanzania?

If yes to #8, move to #9. If no to #8, move to end the interview by following the interview closing script at the bottom of this document.

9. Tell me where you live or have lived in Tanzania, whether mainland or a surrounding territory.
10. What other countries have you lived in?
11. Are you married and how many children do you have? Do you live together?
12. Do you live with anyone who is elderly, ill, or vulnerable to catching COVID-19?
13. How did your family meet its needs during the pandemic?
14. During the pandemic, did you earn money? If so, how did you earn money? If not, why?
15. Before COVID-19, how was your schedule during a typical day?
16. When you learned about COVID-19, did this change your normal activities? If so, share some details about that.
17. What were you doing when you first heard about coronavirus?

18. How were you getting information about what to do during COVID-19? How regularly did you receive information?
19. Did you quarantine or shelter in place? Why did you make that decision?
20. Were you able to use any of your talents, skills, or passions during the pandemic? If so, what are they? If not, why?
21. If COVID-19 disrupted your ability to move and travel, can you share some examples?
22. Did COVID-19 interrupt your ability to be with the community in any way?
23. Did you have to alter any of your or your family's short- or long-term goals as a result of the pandemic? Can you describe those changes?
24. Did being a woman or mother during the coronavirus outbreak impact you differently than it did men?
25. Were you able to access things you as a woman needed during the pandemic? Tell me about that.
26. As a woman or mother, what concerned you most during the pandemic?
27. What about as a Black woman? Did you experience differences in daily life and expectations from other races / non-Black women / tourists?
28. Did you see any differences between daily life and expectations for men and women?
29. Did you know anyone who had COVID-19? Died from COVID-19?
30. How did this experience change your worldview?
31. What was most difficult for you?
32. What gave you hope?
33. During times like these, many people feel powerless, or feel a loss of control. How did you maintain your sense of power and control?

34. Tell me about any beliefs, knowledge, or traditions you held
    before the coronavirus outbreak that helped you during the
    pandemic.

35. For many people, the pandemic was their first experience with
    having to change their day-to-day lives and plans. What advice
    would you give them for surviving and holding on to the idea
    that there is hope for the future?

Additional questions for interviewees who may have been infected
with COVID-19:

1. Can you tell me how you knew you had COVID-19? For example, did you get tested or did you just know because of your
   symptoms?

2. During your recovery, were you on your own, or did you have
   help? Tell me about it.

3. Now that you're recovered, what are you most concerned about?

Thank you for allowing us to interview you for this oral history
project. Only members of the team will have access to the original
interview, which will be stored in a secured location. No identifying
information will be used in any publications. Should you have any
questions, please feel free to reach out to me.[4]

Appendix B: Tanzania in Context

A brief overview of Tanzania's geographic location, economic history,
and encounters with other public health challenges places women's interviews and the government and people's reaction to the COVID-19
pandemic into context. The United Republic of Tanzania is a coastal
country in East Africa well known for its tourism. It's situated on the In-

dian Ocean, south of Kenya and north of Mozambique. The country has an archipelago that includes two islands, Ugunja, better known as Zanzibar, and Pemba. Tourism in mainland Tanzania and Zanzibar Island provide a substantial number of jobs, which improve economic health. Economists Janeth Malleo and Burhan Mtengwa (2018) suggest that the correlation between tourism, gross domestic product, and income serve the country through growth in foreign exchange and currency. Tanzania's future economic growth largely remains dependent on their tourism industry. While Tanzania's former president, Dr. John Magufuli,[5] did not authorize shutdowns to slow the spread of coronavirus, and instead asked Tanzanians to continue their daily lives as normal so the economy would not fail, the immediate removal of tourism due to expatriates and tourists returning home was immediately felt by Tanzanian citizens. Many are supported daily though their interactions with tourists, giving tours, selling souvenirs, doing paid performances, and working in the food industry; it had a lesser negative effect on the federal economy (*The Citizen* 2020b). Many of Magufuli's claims were publicly accepted by community leaders in his proximity, but leaders who have spoken out to reiterate the serious nature of this pandemic have faced government retaliation (*The Citizen* 2020a). How do we begin to assess the ways epidemics, health disparities, and mistrust of Western medicine influence government decision-making during a global crisis, and the consequences these decisions have on Black women?

Notes

1. The names of all women are pseudonyms to protect their identities. Their profiles reflect their circumstances and where they were living at the time of interviews conducted by Amber Walker in December 2020.

2. Writing about the experiences of Black women and the 'Rona in Tanzania calls into question a common tendency to use categories of analysis generated in the context of enslavement and to apply to African subjects

the logic of an African Diaspora that transpired outside of the African continent. Because this volume aims to represent the experiences of Black women and the 'Rona, we must acknowledge that Blackness is not always an identity that women from Tanzania ascribe to themselves. At the same time, Tanzania is home to people of diverse origins, and some do identify as Black women. Owing to this complexity of identity in the Diaspora and on the African continent, this essay identifies women as Black women when they identify as such, and it represents women from Tanzania or Zanzibar as Tanzanian or Zanzibari women. However, it is important to note that by phenotype, all the women interviewed for this essay would be read as Black women in a U.S. context.

3. *Mwairobaini* is Kiswahili for "neem tree." *Airobaini* translates to "forty." The tree is given this name in Tanzania because it is said to cure forty ailments.

4. The documented interview questions do not include follow-up questions asked to further the conversation or for clarification.

5. During the writing of this essay, Dr. John Magufuli died. The vice president announced that his death was due to a heart condition, but others presume it to be COVID-19 (Wamsley and Peralta 2021).

Bibliography

BBC News. 2020. "Coronavirus: John Magufuli Declares Tanzania Free of COVID-19." June 8, 2020. https://www.bbc.com/news/world-africa-529 66016.

The Citizen. 2020a. "Arusha Advocate Albert Msando Arrested over COVID-19 Remarks." April 29, 2020. https://www.thecitizen.co.tz/news/Arusha-advocate -Albert-Msando-arrested-over-COVID-19-remarks/1840340-5538202-xxfl0s /index.html.

———. 2020b. "Magufuli: Our Economy Comes First in COVID-19 Fight." May 17, 2020, https://www.thecitizen.co.tz/news/Magufuli--Our-economy -comes-first-in-COVID-19-fight/1840340-5555628-iu5ti6z/index.html.

Clark, Gracia. 2019. "African Women in the Real Economy: Prehistoric, Precolonial, Colonial, and Contemporary Transitions." In *Holding the World Together: African Women in Changing Perspective*, edited by Nwando Achebe and Claire C. Robertson, 167–89. Madison: University of Wisconsin Press.

Gonzales, Rhonda M., Catherine Cymone Fourshey, and Christine Saidi. 2018. *Bantu Africa: 3500 BCE to Present*. Oxford, U.K.: Oxford University Press.

International Labour Organization. 2021. *Wage and Salaried Workers, Female (% of Female Employment) (Modeled ILO Estimate)*. World Bank. Data retrieved on January 29, 2021. https://data.worldbank.org/indicator/SL.EMP.WORK.FE .ZS?end=2019andmost_recent_year_desc=falseandstart=2019andview=map.

Kottasová, Ivana. 2018. "When Pads Are a Luxury, Getting Your Period Means Missing Out on Life." CNN, October 3, 2018. https://www.cnn.com/2018/10 /03/health/tanzania-period-poverty-asequals-africa-intl/index.html.

Makoni, Munyaradzi. 2021. "Tanzania Refuses COVID-19 Vaccines." *The Lancet* 397, no. 10274 (February): 566. https://doi.org/10.1016/s0140-6736(21)00362-7.

Malleo, Janeth, and Burhan Ahmad Mtengwa. 2018. "Role of Tourism in Tanzania's Economic Development." *International Journal of Academic Research in Economics and Management Sciences* 7, no. 4: 21–31. http://dx.doi.org/10 .6007/IJAREMS/v7-i4/4826.

Mbilinyi, Marjorie J. 1972. "The State of Women in Tanzania." *Canadian Journal of African Studies* 6, no. 2: 371–77. https://doi.org/10.2307/484210.

Nordling, Linda. 2020. "The Pandemic Appears to Have Spared Africa so Far. Scientists Are Struggling to Explain Why." *Science*, August 11, 2020. https:// www.sciencemag.org/news/2020/08/pandemic-appears-have-spared -africa-so-far-scientists-are-struggling-explain-why.

Osseo-Asare, Abena Dove. 2014. *Bitter Roots: The Search for Healing Plants in Africa*. Chicago: University of Chicago Press.

Oyěwùmí, Oyèrónké. 1997. *The Invention of Women: Making an African Sense of Western Gender Discourses*. Minneapolis: University of Minnesota Press.

Poewe, K. O. 1981. *Matrilineal Ideology: Male-Female Dynamics in Luapula, Zambia*. London: Published for the International African Institute by Academic Press.

Saidi, Christine. 2010. *Women's Authority and Society in Early East-Central Africa*. Rochester, NY: University of Rochester Press.

Sippy, Priya. 2021. "Tanzania's New Leader Is Making Up for Lost Time in the Fight Against Covid." *Quartz Africa*, May 7, 2021. https://qz.com /africa/2006013/tanzania-president-samia-hassan-issues-new-covid-19 -restrictions/.

Soy, Anne. 2020. "Coronavirus in Africa: Five Reasons Why Covid-19 Has Been Less Deadly Than Elsewhere." BBC News, October 7, 2020. https://www.bbc .com/news/world-africa-54418613.

Sterner, Judith, and Eugenia W. Herbert. 1995. "Iron, Gender and Power: Rituals of Transformation in African Societies." *African Arts* 28, no. 3 (Summer): 18–19. https://doi.org/10.2307/3337265.

U.S. Embassy Dar es Salaam. 2021. "COVID-19 Information." U.S. Embassy in Tanzania. April 29, 2021. Last updated June 21, 2022. https://tz.usembassy .gov/COVID-19-information/.

Vizenor, Gerald. 2009. *Native Liberty: Natural Reason and Cultural Survivance*. Lincoln: University of Nebraska Press.

Wamsley, Laurel, and Eyder Peralta. 2021. "Tanzanian President John Magufuli, a COVID-19 Skeptic, Has Died." National Public Radio, March 17, 2021. https://www.npr.org/2021/03/17/978336051/tanzania-president-john -magufuli-a-covid-19-skeptic-has-died.

WHO (World Health Organization). 2019. *WHO Global Report on Traditional and Complementary Medicine 2019*. Geneva: World Health Organization. https://apps.who.int/iris/handle/10665/312342.

CHAPTER 5

Exploring Resiliency and Coping Strategies Among Black Women Enrolled in Graduate School During COVID-19 and Overlapping Racial Injustices

Breauna Marie Spencer, Sharnnia Artis, Nitya Mehrotra, Marjorie Shavers, and Stacie LeSure

Introduction

In 2020, the world faced the novel coronavirus disease (COVID-19) pandemic, which affected millions worldwide. Coupled with COVID-19, the United States was met with a second, and ongoing, social crisis: racial injustices. The intersection of COVID-19 and rampant racial injustices have caused a number of barriers and challenges for the Black community (Yancy 2020). For example, Black people have a higher likelihood of being infected with COVID-19 than their white counterparts (Yancy 2020). They also experience psychological health problems due to the continuous killings of Black women and men, which is a result of racial discrimination (Bor et al. 2018; Hassett-Walker 2020). In the midst of COVID-19, there was an increased awareness of racial injustices and killings. These killings have sparked global protests, the Black Lives Matter hashtag has seen an enormous surge on multiple social media platforms, and major companies have donated funds to address police brutality (Maqbool 2020; Beckman 2020; Blankenship and Reeves 2020; Livingston 2020). Additionally, after the video of George Floyd's death became public, the rates of clinical signs of anxiety and depression among Black Americans have increased substantially (Turner and Williams 2020). To be clear, systemic racism and violence against Black people in America is long standing and is not novel, unlike coronavirus.

News outlets have published articles urging the general public to attempt to find some level of normalcy while accommodating COVID-19 limitations (Castin 2020). However, obtaining a sense of normalcy may not be realistic for Black women doctoral students because the term "normalcy" ignores structural issues that continue to hinder their success, such as COVID-19 and overlapping racial injustices. According to a recently published article by *Forbes*, women of color enrolled in doctoral programs during the COVID-19 outbreak face a number of challenges, including psychological stress, difficulty conducting their research projects, and severe isolation and alienation while writing their dissertations and defending their theses virtually while remaining resilient (Chambers 2020). Black women in higher education have encountered a number of educational and social issues in the ivory tower prior to and during COVID-19. Therefore, this study was guided by the following three research questions:

1. How do Black women enrolled in graduate school characterize and perceive their academic experiences while dealing with the effects of COVID-19 and overlapping racial injustices?
2. What does academia look like for Black women in an era of a global pandemic and ongoing racial violence?
3. How can power be reimagined to empower students, especially Black women graduate students?

Black Women's Graduate School Racialized Experiences, Racial Injustices, and Public Health Issues

In general, pursuing a graduate degree program is a complicated process, given the multiple requirements students must successfully complete (Lovitts 2001). When considering the significant role that both race and gender play for women of color, multiple scholars and researchers suggest that Black women graduate students are additionally impacted by systemic racism and sexism, among other formidable social inequalities (Green et al. 2016; Lewis et al. 2016; Willis 2019). For example, Black women enrolled in graduate school typically receive very little academic mentorship and support, which adversely affects their success (Green et al. 2016; Patterson-Stephens, Lane, and Vital 2017). They also experience being the lone Black women in their degree programs, which creates feelings of isolation and alienation, exclusionism, and imposter syndrome in mostly white educational environments (Artis et al. 2018; Johnson-Bailey 2004; Ridgeway et al. 2018).

Overall, some Black women enrolled in graduate degree programs operate within predominately white educational environments. If they attempt to defend themselves against various forms of bias and prejudice in the ivory tower, Black women graduate students are negatively stereotyped (Robinson 2012). Some Black women graduate students cope with the harsh and ever-present realities that shape their educational experiences by opting to mask or conceal certain parts of their social identities; these women also cope by developing strategies to defy the socially constructed stereotypical depictions often scripted onto Black women's bodies (Shavers and Moore 2014).

The review of the current literature presented in this research draws heavily from scholarship published prior to the COVID-19 pandemic. As of the writing of this chapter, there are no current research studies available that have cross-examined Black women's graduate level experiences with COVID-19 and the overlapping, heightened awareness and discussions of systemic racism and racial injustice. Additional research is needed that considers the academic and social experiences of Black women enrolled in graduate school during COVID-19 and overlapping racial injustices. To examine this gap in the literature, qualitative interviews were collected from Black women currently enrolled in graduate school to investigate the academic and social barriers they experience as well as their coping strategies for success during these unprecedented and unpredictable times.

Integrating Black Feminist Thought and Black Women Graduate Students' Experiences

Black Feminist Thought (BFT) serves as the guiding theoretical framework to explore the race-gender experiences of Black women enrolled in graduate school regarding COVID-19 and racial injustices. Overall, BFT was strategically designed to both explore and understand the complex intersectional identities of Black women as well as center the concerns of Black women (Collins 1990). The negative stereotypes that have been applied to Black women are long standing and have adversely impacted their lived experiences (Collins 1990). At the intersection of their Blackness and womanhood, Black women in graduate school endure isolating academic environments, racial discrimination, and unsupportive faculty mentors and peers, on top of contending with negative stereotypes (Green et al. 2016; Joseph 2012; Patterson-Stephens, Lane, and Vital 2017; Robinson 2012). BFT contributes greatly to the field of graduate education because it centers the unique and oftentimes unheard voices of Black women who have been and continue to be oppressed and marginalized in the academy. In this study, we seek to utilize BFT to explore the distinct and intersectional challenges that Black women enrolled in graduate school endure during COVID-19 and overlapping racial injustices.

Methodology

The purpose of this qualitative research study was to examine and understand the experiences of Black women enrolled in graduate school as they attend to their psychological health and well-being, utilizing BFT. The study explores how Black women enrolled in graduate school characterize and perceive their academic experiences and psychological health and well-being while dealing with the effects of COVID-19 and overlapping racial injustices. The Institutional Review Board approved this research prior to data collection, and ethical standards were upheld throughout this study.

Participants

Twenty Black women graduate students in higher education participated in the study. The majority of the participants currently attend predominantly white institutions (PWIs), followed by historically Black colleges and universities (HBCUs). In addition, over 70 percent of all students attended, since the beginning of their education, institutions that offer official online programs; therefore, they did not have to make the transition to online education when most colleges and universities began to close beginning in March 2020. The students who participated in fully online graduate programs selected these programs because it provided them with the flexibility to work full time, raise their families, and take online coursework, which would lessen their commute time as they attempted to maintain a work-life balance. More information about the participants' demographics can be found in table 5.1.

To be eligible for this study, participants had to identify as a Black woman in pursuit of a graduate degree in higher education. Participants were recruited through various email listservs and social media platforms targeting Black women in graduate programs. Snowball sampling was also used to identify additional participants (Patton 2002). Eligible individuals were contacted via email to schedule an interview to take place over Zoom, a video conferencing platform.

The researchers used a criterion-based, purposeful sampling method to target Black women graduate students (Creswell 1998). Purposeful

TABLE 5.1 Demographics of Participants (n=20)

Mean age	35
Academic standing	Full time: 75% (15)
	Part time: 25% (5)
Type of degree program	Doctoral program: 95% (19)
	Master's program: 5% (1)
Format of degree program	Online: 70% (14)
	In person: 15% (3)
	Online with residency requirement: 10% (2)
Mean degree program GPA	3.88
Pell Grant eligible / low income	50% (10)
First-generation college student	45% (9)

sampling was used to allow Black women from graduate programs at PWIs, HBCUs, and Minority-Serving Institutions to provide their unique experiences. The research team interviewed twenty participants to obtain a deep understanding of their complex and multidimensional experiences. Five to twenty-five participants are suggested as an appropriate number of participants in a qualitative study (Creswell 1998). The larger sample size provides comparison among schools, fields, and other individual characteristics and allows for redundancy across participants. Redundancy is a central tenet of qualitative research, indicating that data collection and analysis continue until theoretical saturation or once no new data or concepts of a theory appear (Lewis-Beck, Bryman, and Liao 2003).

Measures

The research team used multiple data sources (e.g., demographic questionnaires, participant interviews, researcher reflection) to triangulate findings and ensure the credibility of the study (Lincoln and Guba 1985). Semi-structured interviews were conducted to address important issues and provide consistency while allowing for flexibility in the participants' responses (Charmaz 2006).

Data Collection

The interviews were collected from October 2020 to November 2020. Each participant received a document with pertinent information regarding the study prior to their interview, which ranged from twenty-five to forty-five minutes. The audio of these interviews was recorded for accurate documentation and was transcribed via Zoom for analysis. After completing the Zoom interviews, participants were emailed a link to a demographic survey. Upon completing both the interview and demographic survey, participants received a $25 Amazon gift card. The interview protocol, which can be found in the appendix to this chapter, contained multiple probing questions to help participants reflect deeply on their experiences as they relate to the research questions.

Data Analysis

Overall, this study used a grounded theory methodological approach. This approach gives researchers the opportunity to generate theory based on the emergence of patterns and themes that are grounded within the findings of the data (Martin and Turner 1986). To analyze the data, our research team read the interview transcripts several times and wrote memos about every participant (Noble and Mitchell 2016). Our research team also analyzed the interview transcripts and created codes that were used to define and categorize the qualitative data accordingly (Charmaz 2012). Short labels were then applied to each interview transcript and a detailed codebook was created to ensure that the data was coded in the same manner across all of the collected data. The codebook consisted of the codes themselves, a short and descriptive definition of each code, and an example. Our research team then culled the list of codes that were originally created by deleting and combining codes in favor of other codes that were more categorically representative. We also compared the findings from the data analysis to the prior literature to explore differences and similarities (Deterding and Waters 2018).

Results and Discussion

This study examined the following research questions:

1. How do Black women enrolled in graduate school characterize and perceive their academic experiences while dealing with the effects of COVID-19 and overlapping racial injustices?
2. What does the institution look like for Black women in an era of a global pandemic and ongoing racial violence?
3. How can power be reimagined to empower students, especially Black women graduate students?

The analysis of the findings revealed two prominent themes based upon the experiences of Black women enrolled in graduate school during the wake of COVID-19 and overlapping racial injustices. Two themes emerged from the data analysis: (1) Where Does My Help Cometh From? My Advisor No Longer Advises Me and Identifying Strategies for Academic and Personal Persistence, and (2) Institutional Care in the Time of COVID-19 and Racial Injustice: Reimagining the Graduate Education Landscape for Black Women.

Where Does My Help Cometh From? My Advisor
No Longer Advises Me and Identifying Strategies for
Academic and Personal Persistence
Many of the Black women in this study discussed a lack of institutional access to adequate academic advising and mentoring from their faculty advisors. As a result, some Black women were left to their own devices to determine how to persist academically as they study and prepare for their comprehensive examinations, identify a thesis topic and defend their proposals, or write their thesis or dissertation. They are also adversely impacted because they have been unable to get in contact with their advisors via email or by telephone in the wake of

the pandemic. In cases where students are able to obtain some level of access to their advisors, this was typically done via email. For example, a student named Ramona recently began her graduate program and she primarily connects with her advisor via email. Ramona clarified, "[My advisor] is very overwhelmed. So [we meet] primarily through email whenever [I] can get in touch with her but it's just [me] trying to figure out [my] schedule on [my] own . . . so it's very challenging but in hindsight I know she is very, very busy." Although Ramona understands that her advisor is very busy, it still causes Ramona to question how she will be able to progress to degree completion without the support of her advisor. She experiences this alongside having to manage being overwhelmed by COVID-19 and overlapping racial injustices.

Another issue that a few of the Black women described is the pre-existing lack of communication they have with their advisors. A student named Charlotte mentioned that she has continuously struggled to effectively communicate with her advisor since prior to COVID-19; Charlotte's level of communication with her advisor has only continued to worsen during the pandemic. Charlotte is currently working on her dissertation proposal and asked her advisor if they could begin meeting weekly because her advisor's feedback was helping her progress in a timely manner. However, as Charlotte recalls, "after we finished the Zoom call . . . I [didn't] hear anything [from my advisor] and I noticed that every time I [asked for help with my research proposal]." Overall, Charlotte's experience has been "really frustrating because I feel like if you want to [be the] chair you [would] support me. Like, why aren't you responding?" Charlotte feels discouraged because her dissertation chair has not acknowledged or responded to her dissertation chapters she sent via email for review and feedback. To date, Charlotte has completed three chapters of her dissertation. Ultimately, she decided to take it upon herself to revise her own dissertation chapters, but at the same time, she is still nervous about whether her dissertation committee will ever respond to her numerous and persistent emails. Hence, students such as Charlotte are under tremendous amounts of stress because they lack institutional support and adequate mentorship. COVID-19 has exacerbated Charlotte's concerns about completing her doctoral program because she is worried "about not getting proper feedback." Therefore, Charlotte worked with a writing specialist and a graduate advisor to obtain the academic support she needs given the long-standing difficult relationship she has with her advisor. Although it can be rather stressful and strenuous to complete a graduate degree program with little to no support, Black women enrolled in graduate school are determined to "finish strong." Black women have acquired these coping strategies to maintain their academic success in the classroom, which includes their psychological health and well-being. The lack of support and mentorship that some of the Black women graduate students have access to also speaks to a lack of institutional accountability.

Regardless of whether or not Black women receive mentorship from their advisors, many have consciously decided to persevere and progress toward degree completion. Another student, Camille, mentioned that she has become "amazingly productive" during COVID-19. In order to cope with the pain associated with George Floyd's death, Camille took to writing. Camille said she was able to write "several papers [that are now] either published or submitted [to academic journals]." However, at the same time, Camille questions herself, stating, "I'm worried about publications and people are dying." Camille understands that she needs to write because it's "therapeutic" in the sense that it gives her the ability to "block out everything in the world." As she attempts to make sense of the current state of the world, Camille repeatedly questions herself for her well-intended actions that center and prioritize her psychological health and well-being. Given Camille's narrative, we are reminded of Audre Lorde's seminal piece "Poetry Is Not A Luxury," which ascribes meaning to the process of writing as a means toward healing. Lorde states, "For women, then, [writing] is not a luxury. It is a vital necessity of our existence. It forms the quality of the light within which we predicate our hopes and dreams toward survival and change, first made it language, then into idea, then into more tangible action" ([1984] 2012, 37). Altogether, Black women must prioritize their self-care without care. In a conversation with the authors over Zoom, Dr. Julia S. Jordan-Zachery conceptualized that Black women must undergo "repair care" due to systemic racism and sexism that they have repeatedly experienced, which is indicative of failing institutional structures and the invisibility of Black women. For Camille, writing is not a luxury because she uses writing as a way to cope and heal given the current state of the world.

Self-care is of vital importance for Black women graduate students to center themselves. To ensure their psychological health and well-being, which includes their physical health, several Black women graduate students decided to put their needs first. In this study, Black women putting their needs first consisted of them exercising, praying, meditating, and listening to their favorite music. These coping strategies are especially needed as they attempt to manage the stress involved in being parents, caregivers, and students, among a host of other titles during the wake of COVID-19 and the overlapping fatalities of Black women and men. The radical self-care that Black women employ in the academy can best be defined by Nicol and Yee:

> [Self-care] involves embracing practices that keep us physically and psychologically healthy and fit, making time to reflect on what matters to us, challenging ourselves to grow, and checking ourselves to grow, and checking ourselves to ensure that we are doing aligns with what matters to us. We consider this self-care "radical" because it fundamentally alters how we make choices about allocating time, money, and energy for ourselves personally, at home, and at work and seeks to revolutionize our workplace practices. Practiced faithfully, "radical self-care" involves owning and directing our lives and choosing with

whom, how, and how often we engage in our nested, interconnected worlds so that we can be unapologetically ourselves in the face of unrelenting pressure and expectations to be otherwise. (2017, 134)

Self-care is a radical act of self-love for many of the students featured in this essay because they want to ensure that they engage in daily practices that will help them to heal. As they reach for some level of normalcy and self-control during these "strange" times, Black women enrolled in graduate school understand that is it important to rest.

These Black women graduate students also believe it important to uplift each other to "finish strong" and graduate. For example, Nelly regularly checks on another Black women enrolled in her graduate program to "just make sure that we're doing okay [and that we are] doing what we need to [be] doing [at work]." Overall, these check-ins for Black women help them because they have someone to talk to, which is especially important since they both operate and exist in predominately white environments where their Blackness and womanhood oftentimes go unnoticed and where there is not much regard for their lived experiences. Thus, having the support of a Black sister helps keep Black women graduate students both encouraged and pressing forward as emerging psychologists, educators, and scientists in their respective disciplines. Black feminism is distinctly rooted in cultivating sisterhood among Black women in order to heal and persevere from a spiritual, psychological, and physical space that uplifts the Black woman and her tribe (Baker-Bell 2017).

Institutional Care in the Time of COVID-19 and Racial Injustice: Reimagining the Graduate Education Landscape for Black Women

Institutional care and concern for Black graduate women is a critical component for cultivating an environment where they thrive in their graduate programs. During a time of COVID-19 and racial injustice, the importance of institutional care has even greater significance. Below are five recommendations, in no particular order, to foster a culture of care for Black graduate women in higher education that is rooted in social justice:

1. Bring awareness to the racism that the Black community faces and create a brave space for people to share their experiences openly

2. Create space for Black graduate women to build community

3. Create time and space for faculty, staff, and students to advocate for causes supporting the Black community

4. Provide cultural competency training

5. Enhance faculty, department, and student accountability

RECOMMENDATION 1: BRING AWARENESS TO THE RACISM THAT THE BLACK COMMUNITY FACES AND CREATE A BRAVE SPACE FOR PEOPLE TO SHARE THEIR EXPERIENCES OPENLY

Black women are multidimensional and bring their various identities to higher education. Their race and gender are identities that cannot be left outside the physical or virtual classroom and laboratory. Current events such as COVID-19, which disproportionately impacts the Black community, and global protests against racism and police brutality are part of Black women's lived experiences that often impact them differently than their non-Black peers, faculty, and staff members (Hayes 2020; Yancy 2020). Given the negative impact of these traumatizing events, it is essential for institutions to bring awareness to racism that the Black community faces and create brave spaces for students, faculty, and staff. Institutions should offer opportunities to have discussions about racism and allow Black and non-Black people to come together to share openly about their experiences.

RECOMMENDATION 2: CREATE SPACE FOR BLACK
GRADUATE WOMEN TO BUILD COMMUNITY
While brave space is recommended to encourage conversations around race, space for Black graduate women to build community with other Black women is just as vital and pivotal. This space is recommended to allow Black women to gather with other women who may share similar backgrounds and experiences.

RECOMMENDATION 3: CREATE TIME AND SPACE FOR
FACULTY, STAFF, AND STUDENTS TO ADVOCATE FOR
CAUSES SUPPORTING THE BLACK COMMUNITY
To combat the racial inequities Black graduate women face, allyship is imperative. Allyship is a process involving listening, confronting systemic racism, and seeking to deconstruct systemic racism. To empower a community of allies and advocates, the institution can host events that provide space for non-Black people to discuss the concerns of the Black community and advocate for causes supporting the Black community. Examples of these types of events could be a town hall, book club, or discussion panel of experts.

RECOMMENDATION 4: PROVIDE CULTURAL
COMPETENCY TRAINING
Given the relative absence of Black women in graduate programs, many non-Black students, faculty, and staff in graduate programs have limited interactions with Black students. Consequently, there is frequently a lack of understanding of the experiences and needs of Black women. To bridge this gap, cultural competency training is recommended to give students, faculty, and staff members the skills they need to understand, work, and succeed interculturally. This training could lead to a better environment and more effective advising and guidance for Black women.

RECOMMENDATION 5: ENHANCE FACULTY, DEPARTMENT, AND STUDENT ACCOUNTABILITY

The harmful and damaging experiences Black women face in their graduate programs are often ignored or remain unaddressed, which is a major issue found within this study. While overt racism and sexism is typically reported and investigated, subtle and more covert racist and sexist acts such as microaggressions tend to be overlooked. Institutions, especially graduate programs, should offer mechanisms for accountability. This could include an anonymous reporting of experiences and climate surveys to understand the perception of students' experiences in the program.

Conclusion: Black Women Graduate Students During the Wake of COVID-19 and Overlapping Racial Injustices

The purpose of this qualitative research study was to examine the academic and psychological experiences of Black women enrolled in graduate school during an unprecedented time. The stressors that Black women graduate students face include a lack of mentorship from their faculty advisors. More specifically, some of the students featured in this essay had not heard from their advisors in the past few weeks or months since the onslaught of COVID-19. Accordingly, Black women are required to rely on themselves, which includes identifying online support via various social media platforms for learning how to study for their comprehensive examinations, develop their dissertation proposals, or write their thesis or dissertation chapters. Some of the students fear that their lack of academic advisement will result in another year being needed to complete their graduate programs or that their advisors will not approve of their thesis or dissertation research studies altogether.

The stressors that Black women encounter in their graduate programs are many. They have to manage their psychological health and well-being because of the associated trauma they experience as it pertains to their racialized and gendered stress. This stress stems from the fact that Black women are required to be strong and resilient. Black women enrolled in graduate school are strong but they are also saddened and depressed by the current state of the world. They question being enrolled in a degree program while the larger Black community is encumbered and afflicted by a pandemic and long-standing racial discrimination. They also question whether attaining their graduate degree will equip them to develop policies and affect change that will help transform the issues that the Black community and other marginalized communities encounter (e.g., discrimination, poverty, police brutality, etc.). Altogether, Black women enrolled in graduate school experience a host of academic and psychological health problems that impede their overall success given COVID-19 and overlapping racial injustices that has resulted in countless deaths of Black people globally.

Acknowledgments

This material is based upon work supported by the National Science Foundation (Award # EEC1648332 and EEC1647986). Any opinions, findings, conclusions, or recommendations expressed in this material are those of the authors and do not necessarily reflect the views of the National Science Foundation.

Appendix: Interview Questions

1. Tell me about yourself and your educational path so far.
2. How would you best describe your academic experiences as a graduate student?

    a. How has that changed since COVID-19?

    b. How does that compare to pre-COVID-19?

    c. How does that compare with the Black Lives Matter social movement?

3. Describe your experiences as a Black woman in your degree program.

    a. How has that changed since COVID-19?

    b. How does that compare with the Black Lives Matter social movement?

4. Where are you at in your degree program? How do you feel about your abilities to complete your coursework, thesis, etc.?

    a. How has that changed since COVID-19?

    b. How does that compare with the Black Lives Matter social movement?

5. How would you describe your relationships with your advisor(s), mentor(s) and peer groups (separate)?

    a. How has that changed since COVID-19? (Additionally probing question: How are you being advised during COVID-19?)

    b. How has this impacted you?

    c. How does that compare with the Black Lives Matter social movement?

6. As a Black woman, describe any challenges (e.g., conflicts, barriers, or discrimination) you have experienced during your degree program.

    a. How did these challenges impact you?

    b. How do you compare these challenges and the impact since COVID-19?

    c. How does that compare with the Black Lives Matter social movement?

7. When you experience challenges in your degree program, what strategies and resources do you use to manage them?

    a. How has that changed since COVID-19?

    b. How does that compare with the Black Lives Matter social
       movement?

8. How would you best describe your psychological health and
   well-being as a student?

    a. How has that changed since COVID-19?

    b. What strategies and resources are you using to manage your
       psychological health and well-being?

    c. How does that compare to pre-COVID-19?

    d. How does that compare with the Black Lives Matter social
       movement?

Bibliography

Artis, Sharnnia, Marjorie C. Shavers, Stacie LeSure, Breauna M. Spencer, and
Aiswarya P. Joshi. 2018. "Re-framing and Reimagining the Doctoral Student Narrative: Black Women's Experiences in Engineering and Computer Science." Paper presented at the 2018 ASEE Annual Conference and Exposition, Salt Lake City, UT, June 2018.

Baker-Bell, April. 2017. "For Loretta: A Black Woman Literacy Scholar's Journey to Prioritizing Self-Preservation and Black Feminist-Womanist Storytelling." *Journal of Literacy Research* 49, no. 4 (October): 526–43. https://doi.org/10.1177/1086296X17733092.

Beckman, Brittany L. 2020. "#BlackLivesMatter Saw Tremendous Growth on Social Media. Now What?" *Mashable SE Asia*, July 2, 2020. https://sea.mashable.com/social-good/11349/blacklivesmatter-saw-tremendous-growth-on-social-media-now-what.

Blankenship, Mary, and Richard V. Reeves. 2020. "From the George Floyd Moment to a Black Lives Matter Movement, in Tweets." *Middle Class Memos* (blog), Brookings Institution. July 10, 2020. https://www.brookings.edu/blog/up-front/2020/07/10/from-the-george-floyd-moment-to-a-black-lives-matter-movement-in-tweets/.

Bor, Jacob, Atheendar S. Venkataramani, David R. Williams, and Alexander C. Tsai. 2018. "Police Killings and Their Spillover Effects on the Mental Health of Black Americans: A Population-Based, Quasi-Experimental Study." *The Lancet* 392, no. 10144 (July): 302–10. https://doi.org/10.1016/S0140-6736(18)31130-9.

Castin, Meredith. 2020. "5 Ways to Find Normalcy in the Times of COVID-19." WebPT (blog). May 18, 2020. https://www.webpt.com/blog/5-ways-to-find -normalcy-in-the-time-of-covid-19/.

Chambers, Brittany. 2020. "13 Doctoral Women of Color: Thriving Amid Missing Graduation Due to COVID-19." *Forbes*. April 14, 2020. https://www .forbes.com/sites/brittanychambers/2020/04/14/13-doctoral-women-of -color-thriving-amid-missing-graduation-due-to-covid-19/#2f84039a79c6.

Charmaz, Kathy. 2006. *Constructing Grounded Theory*. London: Sage Publications.

———. 2012. "The Power and Potential of Grounded Theory." *Medical Sociology Online* 6, no. 3: 2–15.

Collins, Patricia Hill. 1990. *Black Feminist Thought: Knowledge, Consciousness, and the Politics of Empowerment*. New York: Routledge.

Creswell, Jonathan W. 1998. *Qualitative Inquiry and Research Design: Choosing Among Five Traditions*. Thousand Oaks, CA: Sage Publications.

Deterding, Nicole M., and Mary C. Waters. 2018. "Flexible Coding of In-Depth Interviews: A Twenty-First Century Approach." *Sociological Methods and Research* 50, no. 2 (October): 708–39. https://doi.org/10.1177/0049124118 799377.

Green, Dari, Tifanie Pulley, Melinda Jackson, Lori L. Martin, and Kenneth J. Fasching-Varner. 2016. "Mapping the Margins and Searching for Higher Ground: Examining the Marginalization of Black Female Graduate Students at PWIs." *Gender and Education* 30, no. 3 (September): 295–309. https://doi .org/10.1080/09540253.2016.1225009.

Hassett-Walker, Connie. 2020. "George Floyd's Death Reflects the Racist Roots of American Policing." *The Conversation*, June 2, 2020. https://theconver sation.com/george-floyds-death-reflects-the-racist-roots-of-american -policing-139805.

Haynes, Suyin. 2020. "As Protesters Shine a Spotlight on Racial Injustice in America, the Reckoning Is Going Global." *Time*, June 11, 2020. https://time .com/5851879/racial-injustice-protests-europe/.

Johnson-Bailey, Juanita. 2004. "Hitting and Climbing the Proverbial Wall: Participation and Retention Issues for Black Graduate Women." *Race Ethnicity and Education* 7, no. 4 (January): 331–59. https://doi.org/10.1080/13613320 42000303360.

Joseph, Joretta. 2012. "From One Culture to Another: Years One and Two of Graduate School for African American Women in STEM Fields." *International Journal of Doctoral Studies* 7: 125–42. https://doi.org/10.28945/1571.

Lewis, Jioni A., Ruby Mendenhall, Stacy A. Harwood, and Margaret Browne Huntt. 2016. "'Ain't I a Woman?' Perceived Gendered Racial Microaggressions Experienced by Black Women." *Counseling Psychologist* 44, no. 5 (August): 758–80. https://doi.org/10.1177/0011000016641193.

Lewis-Beck, Michael, Alan E. Bryman, and Tim F. Liao. 2003. *The Sage Encyclopedia of Social Science Research Methods*. Thousand Oaks, CA: Sage Publications.

Lincoln, Yvonna S., and Egon G. Guba. 1985. *Naturalistic Inquiry*. Thousand Oaks, CA: Sage Publications.

Livingston, Mercey. 2020. "These Are the Major Brands Donating to the Black Lives Matter Movement. Find Out Where Brands Like Target, Walmart and Facebook Are Donating Right Now." CNET, June 16, 2020. https://www.cnet.com/how-to/companies-donating-black-lives-matter/.

Lorde, Audre. (1984) 2012. "Poetry Is Not a Luxury." In *Sister Outsider: Essays and Speeches*, 36–39. Crossing Press Feminist Series. Trumansburg, NY: Crossing Press. Citations refer to the 2012 edition.

Lovitts, Barbara E. 2001. *Leaving the Ivory Tower: The Causes and Consequences of Departure from Doctoral Study*. Lanham, MD: Rowman and Littlefield.

Maqbool, Aleem. 2020. "Black Lives Matter: From Social Media Post to Global Movement." BBC News, July 9, 2020. https://www.bbc.com/news/world-us-canada-53273381.

Martin, Patricia Y., and Barry A. Turner. 1986. "Grounded Theory and Organizational Research." *Journal of Applied Behavioral Science* 22, no. 2 (April): 141–57. https://doi.org/10.1177/002188638602200207.

Nicol, Donna J., and Jennifer A. Yee. 2017. "'Reclaiming our Time': Women of Color Faculty and Radical Self-Care in the Academy." *Feminist Teacher* 27, no. 2–3: 133–56. https://doi.org/10.5406/femteacher.27.2-3.0133.

Noble, Helen, and Gary Mitchell. 2016. "What Is Grounded Theory?" *Evidence-Based Nursing* 19, no. 2: 34–35. http://dx.doi.org/10.1136/eb-2016-102306.

Patterson-Stephens, Shawna M., Tonisha B. Lane, and Louise M. Vital. 2017. "Black Doctoral Women: Exploring Barriers and Facilitators of Success in Graduate Education." *Higher Education Politics and Economics* 3, no. 1: 157–80. https://doi.org/10.32674/hepe.v3i1.15.

Patton, Lori D., Chayla Haynes, and Natasha N. Croom. 2017. "Centering the Diverse Experiences of Black Women Undergraduates." *NASPA Journal About Women in Higher Education* 10, no. 2: 141–43. https://doi.org/10.1080/19407882.2017.1331627.

Patton, Michael Q. 2002. *Qualitative Research and Evaluation Methods*. Thousand Oaks, CA: Sage Publications.

Ridgeway, Monica L., Ebony O. McGee, Dara E. Naphan-Kingery, and Amanda J. Brockman. 2018. "Black Engineering and Computing Doctoral Students' Peer Interactions That Foster Racial Isolation." Paper presented at the Collaborative Network for Engineering and Computing Diversity Conference (CoNECD), Crystal City, VA, April 2018.

Robinson, Subrina J. 2012. "Spoke Tokenism: Black Women Talking Back About Their Graduate School Experiences." *Race Ethnicity and Education* 16, no. 2: 155–81. https://doi.org/10.1080/13613324.2011.645567.

Shavers, Marjorie C., and James L. Moore III. 2014. "The Double-Edged Sword: Coping and Resiliency Strategies of African American Women Enrolled in Doctoral Programs at Predominately White Institutions." *Frontiers: A Journal of Women Studies* 35, no. 3 (January): 15–38. https://muse.jhu.edu/article/564290.

Tie, Yiona Chun, Melanie Birks, and Karen Francis. 2019. "Grounded Theory Research: A Design Framework for Novice Researchers." *SAGE Open Medicine* 7 (January): 1–8. https://doi.org/10.1177/2050312118822927.

Turner, Erlanger, and Denise Williams. 2020. "Black Americans Experiencing Jump in Rates of Depression, Anxiety After George Floyd Killing." *Washington Post*, June 16, 2020. https://www.washingtonpost.com/health/2020/06/12/mental-health-george-floyd-census/?arc404=true.

Willis, JaQuea M. 2019. "Pushing Through Despite the Bullshit: Black Women Graduate Students in Higher Education at Historically White Institutions." PhD diss., California State University, Long Beach. https://www.proquest.com/docview/2268994480/959E3F4B1B4140F6PQ/1.

Yancy, Clyde W. 2020. "COVID-19 and African Americans." *Journal of the American Medical Association* 323, no. 19: 1891–92. https://doi.10.1001/jama.2020.6548.

CHAPTER 6

Da 'Rona and a Virtual Kitchen Table Politics of Community

Ashley E. Hollingshead and Michelle Meggs

Introduction

I remember going to my grandmother's house as a young girl. Her home, especially during the holidays, was filled with good food, laughter, hugs, affirmations of intellect, and questions about how my siblings and I were doing in school. My grandmother's mantra to me was "Michelle, no man wants a woman with nothing between her ears!" As an educator in the New York City school system, she impressed upon me the importance and necessity of a good education. Also, during our larger family gatherings, amid the raucous laughter between the women and the men, there would be a discussion of politics, good gossip, and good liquor shared between the adults in the room. Her home felt warm and safe. These conversations often moved from the kitchen to the living room, the dining room, and even the piano room. Every area of her home was a space for sharing wisdom, learning family traditions, and remembering those who came before us.

These kitchen table spaces allowed me to imagine a world where Black girls matter, where my brown skin was cherished, where my voice counted, and my soul was nourished in community. With the advent of coronavirus, or da 'Rona, this form of physical and social connection has had to shift. Da 'Rona has taken away the possibility of gathering together in these spaces for respite, refreshment, correction, and reflection. And yet, despite the challenges of da 'Rona and its mandates for social distancing, Black women manage to re-create interstices where they can lay their collective burdens down. Their physical kitchen table gatherings have shifted online, where Black women continue to imagine and create a better future for themselves and their communities.

The kitchen table in Black women's vernacular is the meeting place for intergenerational transmission. Black girls and women gather around kitchen tables to generate, receive, and exchange cultural values and spiritual wisdom (Sampson 2019). The kitchen table is a fluid space, meaning that it can manifest anywhere. Such spaces often tease out an identity politics that recognizes what it means to be both Black and a woman in a society that dishonors both. Black women organize and respond to what Patricia Hill Collins (2002) calls the matrix of domination—race, class, gender, sexual orientation—and how oppression affects Black women. In these spaces, Black women create virtual communities where they challenge and resist harmful hegemonic conversations about Black womanhood and engage in powerful narratives and self-definition. Internet-based communities are digital environments in which individuals, groups, and even organizations interact in virtual (that is to say, nonphysical) spaces (Saunders et al. 2011). In these communities, they engage in similar conversations they had with their grandmothers, aunties, mothers, othermothers, and sisters to talk about life, share home remedies for illnesses, preach the gospel, share good news, and laugh, all while planning how to survive the ravages of racism and sexism (Brown 2000). Here is where Black women continue to resist and persist despite existing in a culture that disregards their voice because of an inability to see their humanity. It is clear that not all women have access to virtual spaces via laptop or desktop computers. However, they may have access through their mobile devices to engage in these online communities. These collectivities fall within the historical trajectory of Black women making room for themselves and doing the work of community building and self-valuation built on a distinct cultural heritage of rejecting discrimination and marginalization. This is evidenced in Black women's activism serving as a point of empowerment for themselves and their communities.

Black women have historically and systematically engaged in reimagining a future where their identities and humanity are honored. The Black women's club movement emerged from Black churches as a counter-discourse to the negative stereotypes placed on Black women and offered a reformulation of Black womanhood (Harris 2003). Black women like Fannie Lou Hamer founded the Mississippi Freedom Democratic Party that challenged an all-white Democratic Party and its lack of representation of all the citizens in the state of Mississippi. Hamer famously testified on national television about the violence she suffered at the hands of law enforcement for registering to vote. Black women engaged in grassroots activism during the civil rights movement through Alabama's Women's Political Council to organize long before the Montgomery bus boycott. The women were not only initiators of action but also sources for spiritual and intellectual empowerment (Crawford et al. 1993). The activism of Black women is a response to their everyday lived realities and as such functions as praxis on how to confront the legacies of sexism, racism, and economic oppression, utilizing the tools available to them. Moreover, their practices continue to build on a blueprint that pushes back against a corrosive system of dominance, manipulation, and exploitation (Taylor 1998) that is fully immersed in white supremacy. Continuing in that lineage of organizing and utilizing modern means of communication, organizations like Until Freedom,[1] cofounded by Tamika Mallory, and communities like Dr. Melva Sampson's Pink Robe Chronicles mobilize people and resources online and in person to respond to the crisis impacting Black and Brown people. There is a recognition that Black people in general, and Black women specifically, have learned to adapt and function in a multiplicity of pandemics. They have worked diligently to make sense of life amid the pandemics of racism, sexism, classism, violence against their bodies, and poverty, just to name a few. No matter the century in which you are born with a "deadly" dose of melanin, or your city of origin, anti-Blackness—among other disenfranchising epistemologies—has and will be an enduring trial (Watkins-Dickerson 2020). Hamer, the Women's Political Council, Mallory, and Sampson envisioned a future where all Black people could take advantage of the promises of American democracy and be recognized as first-class citizens. The creation of online communities as kitchen table gathering spaces falls within and extends this trajectory toward recognition of Black people's subjectivity and humanity.

Dr. Melva Sampson's Pink Robe Chronicles (PRC) community is one of these communities. PRC is an online community that began in response to the death of several Black people, women and men, at the hands of law enforcement. Utilizing a womanist lens, Dr. Melva, as she is called by her followers, calls out the systematic oppression, violence, and racism imposed on Black bodies. Womanism originates from a Black folk expression of "you acting womanish," which usually refers to outrageous, audacious, courageous, or willful behavior (Walker 1983). For Watkins-Dickerson, "womanism begins and ends with the community in which it was born" (2020, 66). She elaborates, "The fundamental markers of womanist work, words, and wisdom are compiled, codified, and cited by the insight, foresight, might, and brightness of everyday Black women who invent reproductions of the everyday horror they survive and thrive beyond, beneath, and beside with a quiet grace and pose. Learning and depending on the words and of women who came before and the women who are yet to come, these Black women build monuments of good measure" (66). Specifically, Dr. Melva speaks truth to power, calls for accountability, and engages in consciousness raising during her Facebook Live videos. This rests in a womanist notion of the power of community to enact change by tapping into the spiritual inheritance of Black people to envision the radical possibility of freedom and traditions of survival.

Dr. Melva's PRC is a womanist response to the ways that systems oppress, depress, and suppress Black bodies and voices. In the age of da 'Rona, while everyone is at risk for contracting the virus, Black and Brown bodies suffer more because of historic inequities regarding access to health care, housing, quality education, and other indicators that measure health outcomes. Black people are dying at 1.7 times the rate of white people from the virus, which means that the toll of the disparities has never been easier to quantify; nineteen thousand Black people would still be alive if not for systemic racism (Peck 2020). PRC stands in the lineage of Black women who respond in a spirit of kinship to the ways that Black life is complicated by the tyranny of white supremacy and its attendant violence. PRC demonstrates how Black women keep "Black womaning" out of the necessity to create landscapes for themselves to make the world around them make sense.

The purpose of this essay is to highlight the ways in which Black women continue to create empowering spaces for themselves in the midst of a pandemic. We will utilize Dr. Melva's PRC community as a case study to highlight how Black women use online spaces to maintain their physical, emotional, and psychological health by focusing on and reimagining holistic self-care through purposeful action and a commitment to caring for one another.

The Pink Robe Chronicles

PRC emerged in 2016, during a complicated and painful time for its founder, Dr. Melva Sampson. Her call to preach was challenged by another Black woman in the church where she was a minister. Dr. Melva's ministry was based on the liberation of Black women, and for a Black woman to say she was not interested in hearing her voice anymore was devastating to her (Benbow 2020). On top of that, the recent and highly publicized (and in some cases, televised) deaths of Eric Garner, Michael Brown, Tamir Rice, Sandra Bland, Philando Castile, and Korryn Gaines at the hands of law enforcement took her grief to another level. In the midst of her heartbreak, Dr. Melva went live on Facebook to try to give language to the unspeakable horror of Black death that kept repeating itself before her eyes. She gave voice to how the intersection of racism, sexism, classism, patriarchy, misogynoir, and homophobia takes aim at Black lives and in one fell swoop eliminates their existence. As a mother, preacher, wife, and Black woman, she went live in her rose-pink robe and honored the names of the dead through the pouring of libations. Dr. Melva did all of this while cooking breakfast at her kitchen table.

The kitchen table became more than her eating space; it became her altar, her pulpit, her sanctuary, and her studio. Here she proclaims the validity, divinity, and absolute humanity of Black life, disrupting a narrative on television that requires Black life to be above reproach in order to be honorable. Dr. Melva uses her online community to have frank conversations with an inclusive—read women, men, LGBTQ+, spiritually fluid—audience to connect around race, gender, sexuality, liberation, and speaking truth to power. Out of this experience, PRC was born. PRC renders visible a womanist praxis of self-awareness and utilizes the kitchen table space as a site of intimate conversation, self-renewal, and self-recovery (Monk-Payton 2020).

In her Facebook Live videos, Dr. Melva is often in her kitchen donning her rose-pink robe. As she greets those who enter her livestream by name, in what she calls her "priestly garments," she engages in the womanist act of communal care. This act eliminates the sense of invisibility and sense of otherness experienced by people who are not white, male, and/or heterosexual. In recognizing each person, she acknowledges and affirms their dignity and humanity, and demonstrates how ordinary Black women are committed to advancing the dignity of all people. Dr. Melva embraces a womanist resistance of being Black, woman, queer, and non-white in the United States, a resistance that thrives without the privileges afforded to white women (Brown 1989). At her kitchen table, Dr. Melva reflects on the lessons of her foremothers, especially those of her maternal grandmother, Annie Inez. Her grandmother's kitchen table was a space where she was introduced to the language of how Black women fight back, talk back, and reclaim their identity in a society that demands their silence and complicity in their oppression. She writes, "Just as Black women's kitchen tables serve as agential sites to combat white supremacy, patriarchy, heterosexism, capitalism, and respectability, social media livestreaming deployed by PRC also becomes an alternative pulpit that affirms the livelihood of all bodies. This is true for bodies that have been sanctimoniously disembodied and dismembered from holy spaces" (Sampson 2019). Black women are honored, and the kitchen table is a site for constructing alternative narratives of wholeness and well-being through lessons learned in these epistemic enclaves.

The kitchen has traditionally been seen as a domestic sphere—where families are nourished with meals prepared by the hands of women. The kitchen space is also where Black women have plotted and planned, from the slave plantation escapes to the civil rights movement to the modern-day Black Lives Matter protests. Set in her kitchen, Dr. Melva transforms a place relegated to meal preparation into a revolutionary space of empowerment, creativity, and advocacy. Around Dr. Melva's virtual kitchen table is where one receives guidance on how to skillfully and creatively resolve life's challenges in the midst of community. In this way, she engages in the womanist act passing on survival skills to subsequent generations.

In a Facebook Live video on January 7, 2017, "Ask for What You Need," Dr. Melva reminds her virtual community about the importance of asking for help. She shares that her grandmother Annie Inez did not model this behavior, and this made it difficult to replicate. Dr. Melva shares that she has since learned that asking for help is not a sign of weakness; in fact, it is a sign of strength because we are supposed to exist in community and depend on it. Asking for help should happen at the table. It seems like a simple lesson, but non-white people in general, and non-white women in particular, have learned that asking for help—directions or clarity—could have challenging or deadly consequences. Nevertheless, Dr. Melva urges her followers to build trust that the community can hold their collective truths and envision the radical possibilities of communal making, even in digital spaces. In offering this truth, Dr. Melva critiques how kitchen spaces attempt to limit women as simply purveyors of meals and physical sustenance. Utilizing her kitchen space, she offers "food" that sustains intellectually, spiritually, and emotionally. In this way, she contributes to consciousness raising by developing resilient communities both on- and offline. Words are not enough to develop these communities. What is needed is an investment of resources needed to break interlocking cycles of oppression. This is representative of how Black women survive, thrive, and flourish.

Womanism regards Black women as more committed to the eradication of the tyranny of oppression and to social justice in comparison to white women. It examines the underlying power dynamics that lead to Black women being perceived as object rather than subject in a white patriarchal culture. Womanism centers Black women's agency as essential rather than an afterthought or peripheral, as in white feminist thought. Black women's ways of knowing and agency are thus prioritized (Smith 2018). Womanism takes place within the daily cycle of life and relies on common solutions to everyday problems. Dr. Melva came on one of her livestreams to announce the founding of the Ubuntu Collective.[2] *Ubuntu* generally means "I am because you are." It points to a worldview based on core values of well-being, flourishing, reciprocal solidarity, and humanity's cooperation to ensure the thriving of everyone (Karenga 2014). It is a recognition that we are all connected and what happens to one happens to all. The purpose of the Ubuntu Collective was to respond to families in need during the pandemic. Those who were part of the PRC community were asked, if they felt led to do so, to contribute $100 per month, or whatever they could afford, to support at least three households for six months headed by single mothers who had lost their jobs because of the COVID-19 pandemic. This is the kind of help that Black women engage in around the kitchen table in person—a form of mutual aid that gathers together needed resources to help others who are suffering. Black women's historical legacy of economic deprivation and their genius of making a way out of no way contributes to their survival wisdom (Phillips 2006). PRC and the Ubuntu Collective fall within the genealogy of mutual aid and benevolent societies that provided support in times of crisis. As the comments bubbling up in the chat showed, people quickly responded to the call for help; some were able to commit to $100 and others to smaller amounts. In the end, PRC and the Ubuntu Collective were able to support six single-parent families for six months early in the pandemic. This is an example of how the virtual kitchen table remains a space for Black women's community building, organizing, caretaking, and a commitment to social justice in the midst of a crisis.

The Time for Kitchen Tables Is Now: Caretaking and Violence During da 'Rona

Essential Work Equals Economic Exploitation
and, Maybe, Death from da 'Rona

COVID-19, a highly infectious airborne disease, has spread globally. U.S. counties with a significant Black population have had higher transmission and death rates compared to other counties (Oppel et al. 2020). In the past year, the United States enacted periods of lockdowns, forcing businesses and other places of employment to close or limit occupancy for indeterminate amounts of time. In the first few months of the pandemic, 41 percent of Black businesses closed due to COVID-19 (Brooks 2020). Lockdowns also create the perfect conditions for emotional and psychological distress to afflict an already vulnerable population, as they prevent physical and intimate interactions with friends and loved ones (SAMHSA 2020). For Black women, their principal and assumed roles as caretakers and their overrepresentation in low-wage essential work create additional barriers to navigating the new realities presented by the pandemic. In the face of evolving forms of violence during da 'Rona, virtual spaces like PRC ensure Black women are cared for.

Historically, racial, gendered, and classed biases produce structural inequalities that limit Black women's access to job opportunities and financial security. Race and gender played a vital role in relegating Black women to low-paid domestic work in the late nineteenth and early twentieth centuries, as employers preferred to hire white and Black men over women for high-wage positions, under the assumption that men were the primary earners for their families (Harley 1990). Current statistics reflect Black women's continued overrepresentation in domestic and service work, particularly in jobs that support life in their community, such as nurses, nursing assistants, home health aides, and elementary and middle school teachers (Kassa and Wilson 2020). Domestic and service work that include face-to-face interactions is now considered "essential work," work that is required to maintain critical infrastructure or to maintain human life (Kassa and Wilson 2020). Overrepresented in essential work, Black women are now faced with the choice of exposing themselves to the virus or financial strain if they decide not to work.

Despite Black women's extensive participation in positions considered essential, they receive less compensation and are more susceptible to losing their jobs compared to white males in similar fields. For instance, Black women make 11 to 27 percent less than their white male counterparts (Kassa and Wilson 2020). Furthermore, during the pandemic, employers are cutting service jobs occupied by Black and Latinx women at disproportionate rates (Kurtz 2021). With few job prospects during the pandemic, the flexibility to leave jobs is stunted, thereby exacerbating Black women's exposure to the virus. Consequently, Black women's communal networks are at higher risk, leading to much fewer of the face-to-face interactions that are significant for community sustenance. Economic precarity leaves an array of psychological and emotional consequences for Black women—we should pay attention to these consequences not just in the short term but with an eye to the longer-term impacts.

Black Women's Lives Matter: Violence Against Our Bodies, Our Lives

Black women are crucial members of their communities, serving as othermothers, financial providers, and a listening ear. Their presence ensures that community members thrive in the face of limited institutional support. However, Black women are also exposed to the dangers of community, as they are more likely to observe and experience physical violence in their neighborhoods than in a different neighborhood (Jenkins 2002; Davis 2012). Black women are also disproportionately vulnerable to several forms of intimate partner violence, including physical violence, sexual violence, and economic exploitation (Richie 2012). Additionally, Black women are vulnerable to state-sanctioned and gendered violence in their communities.

Regardless of age, Black women and girls face violence. Consider that Black girls and young women between the ages of fourteen and twenty-four are also prone to witness or experience police violence in their neighborhoods (Hitchens, Carr, and Clampet-Lundquist 2018). Black cis and trans women are often underdiscussed victims of police violence, even though research denotes Black cisgender and transgender women are also subject to police harassment (Richie 2012;

Crenshaw et al. 2015; Transgender Law Center n.d.). Exposure to violence is proven to spur psychological distress, accelerate the deterioration of physical health, and produce desensitization to violence (Jenkins 2002). In communities of color, where police harassment is widespread, da 'Rona creates new opportunities for police harassment and surveillance. For example, within the first few weeks of the pandemic, police data in New York City indicated that law enforcement disproportionately used distance-enforcement strategies in communities of color (Bates 2020). With limited mobility and an increased police presence in communities of color, Black women are vulnerable to police harassment and communal violence.

Black women are uniquely situated within overlapping systems of oppression and marginalization, which hinders Black women's ability to maintain spaces that provide support. Da 'Rona threatens Black women's safety and livelihood inside and outside of their communities, exacerbating already-unfavorable conditions in the spaces they inhabit. As the current pandemic limits mobility, people are mostly confined to their homes and neighborhoods, preventing interactions with larger communal networks and spaces that provide safety and healing. While interactions with community members can spur the physical and emotional bonds necessary during the pandemic, those interactions can also leave Black women more vulnerable to gendered violence. Furthermore, increased time in the home without access to safe spaces and close friends and family leaves more Black women vulnerable to gendered violence in the home. There is an increased need for Black women to provide emotional and financial support during the pandemic. As a response, Black women shift to online spaces to navigate the challenges presented by da 'Rona. Virtual kitchen tables like PRC are aware of the precarity of this moment. Da 'Rona intensifies issues already present in Black communities, allowing PRC to continue the work it has always done to address the series of hardships Black women experience, and to provide the additional emotional and material tools Black women need to maintain their livelihoods during this unprecedented time. PRC's tenet of communal care guarantees conversations on police violence, economic vulnerabilities, and mental health are front and center.

Theorizing Black Women's Use of the Kitchen Table

What does PRC tell us about Black women's use of the kitchen table? In a society that is openly hostile toward and refuses to accept the full humanity of Black women, the kitchen table operates as a place where Black women gather to adequately address their needs and redefine their Black womanhood. The kitchen table points to the racism, patriarchy, and class oppression Black women face. It becomes a literal and figurative site of activism, where Black women redefine positions of power and shift toward more egalitarian modes of operating. This movement toward egalitarianism and equity becomes a powerful tool for reimagining, reconstructing, and transforming societal norms (Westfield 2009). As Dr. Layli Maparyan (formerly Phillips) asserts, "The kitchen table is an informal, woman-centered space where all are welcome and all can participate. The table is an invitation to become part of a group . . . people can come and go, agree or disagree, take turns talking or speaking all at once, and laugh, shout, complain, or counsel—even be present in silence. It is a space where the language is accessible and the ambiance is casual. At the kitchen table, people share the truths of their lives on equal footing and learn through face-to-face conversation" (Phillips 2006). Through this transformation of space, we witness what Westfield calls a "concealed gathering," where Black women provide hospitality to themselves and each other for resilience (2009, 319). The kitchen table engages in work that promotes healing, equity, and justice for everyone seated there.

At the kitchen table, Black women's collective humanity is recognized, emphasizing the everyday experiences of Black women that need attention. The kitchen table as a womanist space grants epistemological privilege to the lived everyday realities of Black women. Doing so reclaims the interstices necessary to overcome subordination (Floyd-Thomas 1999, 4). This kind of womanist resistance becomes possible when Black women are willing to act courageously and willfully to eradicate oppression. The politics of fear, hatred, and division are rejected at the kitchen table, where instead empowerment, affirmation, and collaboration are cherished.

The kitchen table remains a critical space for Black women, as Black women are always in need of spaces that resist dominant structures of oppression. In a society that is constantly shifting, new structures reinforcing patriarchal norms continuously threaten the livelihood of Black women, attempting to keep Black women at the margins. To combat tyrannical structures, Black women engage in a kitchen table politics, deliberately placing Black women in a position of authority, giving a voice to their needs and desires. Black women acknowledge the commonality of intersectional experiences that exist around race, gender, and class oppression. Placing Black women's politics at the center emerges out of a need to hold accountable those who prevent Black women's access to power. Through this reorientation, the conversations around the table become classrooms where women learn how to recognize and respond to oppression (Westfield 2009). These spaces are not designed to hide from the world but are necessary to engage in revolutionary and transformative actions that build resilient girls, women, and communities.

A Virtual Kitchen Table

As the kitchen table as a cultural site moves beyond the physical realm, online communities like PRC are answering the call to form necessary spaces for Black women to congregate and galvanize. Feeling safe, seen, and supported is especially important in the age of da 'Rona. Virtual kitchen tables serve as nonphysical spaces where Black women maintain their agency as they gather to break down the gendered dynamics of spaces that conform to heteropatriarchy. Virtual kitchen tables bypass traditional biases that discourage certain populations from entering communal spaces, including but not limited to classism, ableism, sexism, ageism, homophobia, and transphobia. Circumventing historical barriers to needed spaces allows for the possibility of equal representation and participation in online spaces, sparking a shift in traditional discourse and domination. Here Black women maintain their physical, psychological, and emotional health. Black women continue the tradition of creating spaces when they are unavailable. As the primary voices in this tradition, Black women maintain their autonomy in public, yet confined, spaces (Collins 1998).

The virtual kitchen table offers Black women a space to express their desires and delineate their needs. What emerges is a virtual kitchen table politics that conveys the concerns of everyday Black women and what they confront daily. This politics is a response to how oppression renders Black women invisible, reduced to problematic binaries, and marginalized. The politics of the virtual kitchen table means that Black women have another avenue to get clear about their identities and how they define themselves. As they walk in many intersectionalities, these spaces make room for all women. Difficult conversations and disagreements are a guarantee, yet those discussions open the pathway to understanding another perspective rather than promoting division. An emerging virtual kitchen table politics facilitates the survival of all Black women.

Online kitchen tables can reach a wide range of audiences, yet they also have the potential to encounter similar barriers that discourage Black communities and Black women from engaging in transformative discourse. The public nature of online spaces can provide access to voices that may not agree nor see the value of those spaces (Steele 2018). Access to and mastery of social networking platforms require both financial resources and technological savvy that are not afforded to everyone. Online platforms can also pressure participants to perform outside their authentic selves, promoting discourse that does not address the needs of their minds, bodies, and spirits (Steele 2018). However, the curated nature of online kitchen tables encourages authenticity and mitigates harmful interactions for those who are most vulnerable (Steele 2018; Sampson 2019). These spaces establish themselves as intimate spaces where members are granted the opportunity to adequately express their frustrations and foster exchanges that attend to their bodily and spiritual desires.

Black online communities have long curated kitchen tables on online platforms, such as blogs, Zoom, Twitter, Facebook, Instagram, etc., to create strategies that provide much-needed resources and foster resistance to commonly held gendered norms (Steele 2018; Sampson 2019). PRC's use of online platforms, as aforementioned, fosters community, provides resources to community members, and challenges oppressive structures. Other Black women have also relied on online platforms to develop community and provide assistance to others. Candice Benbow used her online platforms to raise money for women who could not afford groceries. She also began to use her Instagram Live sessions to discuss motherhood, spirituality, and body politics, reminding Black women to lean on grace and self-love as Black women experience emotional exhaustion during the pandemic. A community of Black women, including Rachel Elizabeth Cargle on Instagram and Twitter and Alex Elle on Instagram, provide space on their online platforms to have discussions with Black women on issues surrounding the mind, body, and spirit.[3]

The drastic and sudden shifts in everyday realities spurred by da 'Rona provide the pathway for Black women to develop kitchen tables in online spaces. The presence of a highly contagious virus has far-reaching consequences for Black communities and Black women. However, by engaging in kitchen table politics, Black women press on to develop more expansive and more inclusive "tables" for them to lean on to navigate new and evolved threats. As the pandemic continues, Black women have used their platforms to focus on the holistic care of Black women's minds, bodies, and spirits. PRC fosters Black women's well-being in this tradition.

Conclusion

Da 'Rona remains a villainous public health threat. It continues to exacerbate the economic, social, and emotional crisis of this country. The virus highlights ever-expanding disparities that increasingly punish communities of color at alarming rates. Virtual kitchen table communities are necessary and critical spaces for Black women in times such as these. They are sustainable, resource-building places where Black women hold space for themselves and others because they understand that no one else will. These gathering spaces are fluid and work to construct strategies for resilience during da 'Rona and beyond. Virtual kitchen tables in the age of da 'Rona are where Black women make inconceivable strides for the survival of self and for the entire race. Virtual kitchen table spaces exist as alternative mechanisms of support in the midst of the pandemic. Here Black women do the necessary work of maintaining their physical, psychological, and emotional health by asking for help, providing mutual aid, and engaging in consciousness raising. Moreover, as these virtual kitchen tables become places of renewal, they also become sites of creativity, advocacy, and action. Dr. Melva Sampson's PRC is an example of how Black women, in moments of struggle against domination, oppression, and the violence of white supremacy, create spaces where they can find joy, respite, and a place to celebrate the beauty of themselves despite the circumstances.

Notes

1. According to their website, Until Freedom is an intersectional social justice organization rooted in the leadership of diverse people of color to address systemic racial injustice. Until Freedom focuses on investing in those people and communities who are most directly impacted by cyclical poverty, inequality, and state violence. They are a clearinghouse for advocates, new and budding activists, seasoned community organizers, students, movement lawyers, entertainers and artists, policy experts, formerly and currently incarcerated individuals, and survivors of gun violence to work linearly to uplift all of our people. For more information about Until Freedom, please visit https://untilfreedom.com/about/.

2. The Ubuntu Collective was a temporary COVID relief effort to aid families during the pandemic. The PRC community may activate this effort as needed to meet the need of individuals and families with emergency needs.

3. For more information on Rachel Elizabeth Cargle and Alex Elle, please visit @rachel.cargle and @alex on Instagram.

Bibliography

Bates, Josiah. 2020. "Police Data Reveals Stark Racial Discrepancies in Social Distancing Enforcement Across New York City." *Time*, May 8, 2020. https://time.com/5834414/nypd-social-distancing-arrest-data.

Benbow, Candice. 2020. "While More Black Churches Come Online Due to Coronavirus, Black Women Faith Leaders Have Always Been Here." *Essence*, March 24, 2020. https://www.essence.com/feature/more-black-churches-online-coronavirus-black-women-faith-leaders-always-been-here/.

Brock, André. 2009. "'Who Do You Think You Are?' Race, Representation, and Cultural Rhetorics in Online Spaces." *Poroi* 6, no. 1: 15–35. https://doi.org/10.13008/2151-2957.1013.

Brooks, Rodney A. 2020. "More Than Half of Black-Owned Businesses May Not Survive COVID-19." *National Geographic*, July 17, 2020. https://www.nationalgeographic.com/history/article/black-owned-businesses-may-not-survive-covid-19.

Brown, Kelly Delaine. 1989. "God Is as Christ Does: Toward a Womanist Theology." *Journal of Religious Thought* 46, no. 1 (Summer): 7–16.

Brown, Teresa L. Fry. 2000. *God Don't Like Ugly: African American Women Handing on Spiritual Values*. Nashville: Abingdon Press.

Collins, Patricia Hill. 1998. *Fighting Words: Black Women and the Search for Justice.* Minneapolis: University of Minnesota Press.

——. 2002. *Black Feminist Thought: Knowledge, Consciousness, and the Politics of Empowerment.* New York: Routledge.

Crawford, Vicki L., Jacqueline Anne Rouse, Barbara Woods, and Broadus Butler, eds. 1993. *Women in the Civil Rights Movement: Trailblazers and Torchbearers, 1941–1965.* Bloomington: Indiana University Press.

Crenshaw, Kimberlé, Andrea Ritchie, Rachel Anspach, Rachel Gilmer, and Luke Harris. 2015. *Say Her Name: Resisting Police Brutality Against Black Women.* New York: African American Policy Forum.

Davis, Dána-Ain. 2012. *Battered Black Women and Welfare Reform: Between a Rock and a Hard Place.* Albany: State University of New York Press.

Floyd-Thomas, Stacey M. 1999. "Introduction: Writing for Our Lives— Womanism as an Epistemological Revolution." *Deeper Shades of Purple: Womanism in Society and Religion,* edited by Stacey M. Floyd-Thomas, 1–16. New York: New York University Press.

Gould, Elise, and Valerie Wilson. 2020. *Black Workers Face Two of the Most Lethal Preexisting Conditions for Coronavirus—Racism and Economic Inequality.* Washington, D.C.: Economic Policy Institute, June 1, 2020. https://www.epi.org/publication/black-workers-covid/.

Harley, Sharon. 1990. "For the Good of Family and Race: Gender, Work, and Domestic Roles in the Black Community, 1880–1930." *Signs: Journal of Women in Culture and Society* 15, no. 2 (Winter): 336–49. http://www.jstor.org/stable/3174489.

Harris, Paisley Jane. 2003. "Gatekeeping and Remaking: The Politics of Respectability in African American Women's History and Black Feminism." *Journal of Women's History* 15, no. 1 (Spring): 212–20. https://doi.org/10.1353/jowh.2003.0025.

Hitchens, Brooklynn K., Patrick J. Carr, and Susan Clampet-Lundquist. 2018. "The Context for Legal Cynicism: Urban Young Women's Experiences with Policing in Low-Income, High-Crime Neighborhoods." *Race and Justice* 8, no. 1 (January): 27–50. https://doi.org/10.1177%2F2153368717724506.

Jenkins, Esther J. 2002. "Black Women and Community Violence: Trauma, Grief, and Coping." *Women and Therapy* 25, no. 3–4: 29–44. https://doi.org/10.1300/J015v25n03_03.

Karenga, Maulana. 2014. "Nommo, Kawaida, and Communicative Practice." In *The Global Intercultural Communication Reader,* edited by Molefi Kete Asante, Yoshitaka Miike, and Jing Yin, 211–25. New York: Routledge.

Kassa, Melat, and Valerie Wilson. 2020. "Black Women Workers Are Essential During the Crisis and for the Recovery but Still Are Greatly Underpaid." Economic Policy Institute, August 12, 2020. https://www.epi.org/blog/black-women-workers-are-essential-during-the-crisis-and-for-the-recovery-but-still-are-greatly-underpaid/.

Kurtz, Annalyn. 2021. "The US Economy Lost 140,000 Jobs in December. All of Them Were Held by Women." CNN Business, January 8, 2021. https://www.cnn.com/2021/01/08/economy/women-job-losses-pandemic/index.html.

Monk-Payton, Brandy. 2020. "Staging Womanist Visibility on *Red Table Talk*." *Women's Studies in Communication* 43, no. 4: 1–8. https://doi.org/10.1080/07491409.2020.1831867.

Oppel, Richard A., Robert Gebeloff, K. K. Rebecca Lai, Will Wright, and Mitch Smith. 2020. "The Fullest Look Yet at the Racial Inequity of Coronavirus." *New York Times*, July 5, 2020. https://www.nytimes.com/interactive/2020/07/05/us/coronavirus-latinos-african-americans-cdc-data.html.

Peck, Patrice. 2020. "The Virus Is Showing Black People What They Knew All Along." *Atlantic*, December 22, 2020. https://www.theatlantic.com/health/archive/2020/12/pandemic-black-death-toll-racism/617460/.

Phillips, Layli, ed. 2006. *The Womanist Reader*. New York: Taylor and Francis.

Richie, Beth. 2012. *Arrested Justice: Black Women, Violence, and America's Prison Nation*. New York: New York University Press.

SAMHSA (Substance Abuse and Mental Health Services Administration). 2021. *Double Jeopardy: COVID-19 and Behavioral Health Disparities for Black and Latino Communities in the U.S.* Rockville, MD: SAMHSA, January 1, 2021. https://www.samhsa.gov/sites/default/files/covid19-behavioral-health-disparities-black-latino-communities.pdf.

Sampson, Melva. 2019. "Going Live: The Making of Digital Griots and Cyber Assemblies." *Practical Matters Journal* 12 (Summer): 10–30. http://practicalmattersjournal.org/2019/10/16/going-live-the-making-of-digital-griots-and-cyber-assemblies/.

Saunders, Carol, Anne F. Rutkowski, Michiel Genuchten van, Doug Vogel, and Julio Molina Orrego. 2011. "Virtual Space and Place: Theory and Test." *MIS Quarterly* 35, no. 4 (December): 1079–98. https://doi.org/10.2307/41409974.

Sheared, Vanessa. 2006. "Giving Voice: An Inclusive Model of Instruction: A Womanist Perspective." In *The Womanist Reader*, edited by Layli Phillips, 269–79. New York: Taylor and Francis.

Smith, Mitzi J. 2018. *Womanist Sass and Talk Back: Social (In)Justice, Intersectionality, and Biblical Interpretation*. Eugene, OR: Cascade Books.

Steele, Catherine Knight. 2018. "Black Bloggers and Their Varied Publics: The Everyday Politics of Black Discourse Online." *Television and New Media* 19, no. 2 (May): 112–27. https://doi.org/10.1177%2F1527476417709535.

Taylor, Ula Y. 1998. "Making Waves: The Theory and Practice of Black Feminism." *Black Scholar* 28, no. 2 (Summer): 18–28. https://doi.org/10.1080/000 64246.1998.11430912.

Transgender Law Center. n.d. "Prisons and Policing Resources." Accessed August 7, 2022. https://transgenderlawcenter.org/resources/prisons.

Walker, Alice. 1983. *In Search of Our Mothers' Gardens: Womanist Prose.* New York: Harvest.

Watkins-Dickerson, Dianna. 2020. "'Don't Get Weary': Using a Womanist Rhetorical Imaginary to Curate the Beloved Community in Times of Rhetorical Emergency." *Journal of Communication and Religion* 43, no. 3 (Autumn): 62–74. https://www.academia.edu/44789570/_Dont_Get_Weary_Using_a _Womanist_Rhetorical_Imaginary_to_Curate_the_Beloved_Community_in _Times_of_Rhetorical_Emergency.

Westfield, Lynne. 2009. "She Put Her Foot in the Pot: Table Fellowship as a Practice of Political Activism." *Creating Ourselves: African Americans and Hispanic Americans on Popular Culture and Religious Expression*, edited by Anthony B. Pinn and Benjamín Valentín, 339–55. Durham, NC: Duke University Press.

CHAPTER 7

Black Motherschooling

Creating a Liberatory Community for Home Education

Candace S. Brown, Kaja Dunn, Kendra Jason,
Janaka B. Lewis, and Tehia Starker Glass

Introduction

The first case of coronavirus disease 2019 (COVID-19) in North Carolina was diagnosed on March 3, 2020. By March 10, North Carolina had declared a state of emergency to coordinate health, safety, and welfare efforts in response to COVID-19. On March 16, Governor Roy Cooper ordered K–12 schools to close and on March 17 signed an executive order to broaden unemployment benefits as businesses, workplaces, and community organizations closed indefinitely.[1] As five Black women, mothers, and scholars in fields across humanities, health, social sciences, education, and performance arts (a.k.a. sisterscholars), the closure of both the university and the schools our children attended resulted in additional pressure on stressors already present for Black women faculty members (Williams and Hardaway 2018). Pressure to continue the pillars of work (i.e., teaching, research, service) for tenure and promotion while being fully present for our now-stay-at-home children's personal and academic needs caused an already off-kilter work-life balance to come completely unhinged.

Home, the safe haven away from our demanding jobs, dissipated, and the lines of work and home blurred. The hours of school, work, and home life extended into sleeping hours. The expectations of increased performance and presence in online meetings became overwhelming. Additionally, the murders of Ahmaud Arbery (February 23), Breonna Taylor (March 13), George Floyd (May 25), Tony McDade (May 27), and countless others named and unnamed added an additional toll on our souls. As we have done historically, and now in the present time, we, as Black mothers, banded together to take care of one another, support one another, and manage all of the catastrophes and keep ourselves and our families intact (Berry and Gross 2020).

Motherschooling as an Act of Resistance for Black Mothers

"Homeschooling" in a pandemic is not the same as a homeschool community where families choose to educate their children at home with an approved curriculum external to the school system. We, instead, based our approach in the idea of motherscholars, which originates from Matias's critical race parenting, defined as "an educational praxis that can engage both parent and child in a mutual process of teaching and learning about race, especially ones that debunk dominant messages about race" (2016, 3). However, what we do is beyond that of a motherscholar, the work of which we see as individual in nature. What we refer to as motherschooling is a collective approach to the ways we raise our children, protect their racial identity, and maintain all of our joy. Through motherschooling, joy is a form of resistance in the face of oppression that exists in our worlds. At the heart of motherschooling is resistance, liberation, and joy. Because we school in community, motherschooling is the sentiment of managing both home and work life, and now includes the schooling of our children. We practice motherschooling in the ways *we are in community with one another*, our community, and our families.

Although we already knew one another through our university, we bonded through the process of motherschooling during the pandemic outbreak of 2020. Motherschooling became a normative practice in our homes and with each other. We used Black-owned curriculum companies, or modified the "standard curriculum," to center Blackness within a specialized set of educational materials for our children to exchange. We designed and engaged in extracurricular learning activities as a group. We built lessons to do with our children as we celebrated Juneteenth and the Fourth of July, and experienced the negative results of the racial injustices of our country. Some of our children who were similar in age were playmates and classmates in our homes. Our children were all fully engaged in public and private school systems, supplemented by motherschooling of our own design and implementation of curriculum. While the demands of our jobs were greater, we had more options for and more control of our children's education.

Although we experienced raising Black children in public and private educational systems that did not fully support their needs, in spite of our best intentions, none of us were fully prepared for the ways that COVID-19, or the 'Rona, would fully challenge and transform the model of "business as usual" for any of our families. In the ancestral tradition of collective and collaborative formation of "teaching to transgress," as bell hooks (1994) discusses in her book of that name, we created an educational homespace for our children in addition to the homeplace they already experienced. Motherschooling became the intervention that allowed us to go beyond simply schooling at home to choosing what we wanted to instill in our children.

Across five different disciplines—education, English literature, health, theatre, and sociology, which shaped our individual and collective methodologies—we decided that we did not want to do the work of scholarship or teaching our children by ourselves. More than just working from home (for them and for us), motherschooling was a way to curate their educational experiences in response to what they faced outside of our homes. In her essay, "BlackGirlMagic Is Real," Tammy Owens states, "The ingenuity and creativity of Black girls and women have been invaluable to American culture. Yet, the terms *genius* or *innovator* or others, such as *intellectual* and *theorist*, are rarely attributed to Black women and girls" (2019, 185). Instinctively, sister-scholars reached across disciplines, pooled intellectual (and often-times physical) resources, created space for support, problem-solved, mourned, listened, and celebrated. While the world burned around us, and then demanded we answer its calls, texts, and emails about racism and how to address it, we found ways to breathe with each other.

We are fully aware of the ways we, as Black mothers, are consistently teaching our children about race and constantly empowering them in conversation and daily activities. While the world is slowly discovering the efficacy of Black women, it remains wholly unaware of the resourcefulness and power of Black mothers. This pandemic exposed the *secret power of Black motherhood*: a lifetime of operating on the margins, in spaces not built for us—as Black people, as women, as mothers—has led to a *skill set of quickly maneuvering, innovating, rethinking, adjusting, and surviving*. As with many Black mothers inside and outside of the academy, this developed skill of "navigating the margins" proved invaluable as we also guided our children through "sheltering in place."

This essay collaboration of multi-ethnographic methods (to draw from Roby and Cook's 2019 discussion of duo-ethnography) was derived from community thinking, support, and shared resources. Although we were practicing these educational methods with our children before, working together has influenced how we think about our children's educational and interactional experiences with the U.S. school system and further encouraged us to build the brilliance of Blackness in home education. We are not alone. Our five voices represent a larger dialogue burgeoning in the Black community. Since the onslaught of the dual pandemics of violence against Blackness and COVID-19, we have also witnessed the increasing influence of Black media and journalism (e.g., the 1619 Project, Verzuz TV, Black Twitter, vegan Tabitha Brown's platforms), Black communities (e.g., the creation of Freedom, Georgia), Black-centered policy (e.g., the Biden administration's Executive Order 13985, Advancing Racial Equity and Support for Underserved Communities Through the Federal Government), corporate advocacy for Black Lives Matter (e.g., the creation of anti-racist policies), Black businesses, and Black education networks (e.g., the Abolitionist Teaching Network and the Sankofa Club) on the larger American society.

Black feminist author, educator, scholar, and activist Dr. Anna Julia Cooper stated, "A stream cannot rise higher than its source" ([1892] 1988, 29). The irony is not lost on us that we were designated as our children's primary educators during their shift of learning methods while, at the same time, our academic positions demanded more. We tried to continue to find a healthy space between our positions as parents and as professors. Our children's education is not our primary occupation, but we tried to create an educational support network for the shift they experienced. Motherschooling allowed our voices to be heard by recentering the ideas of Black women and Black motherhood, brought from an "othered" subgroup (both as Black women and as mothers who are Black women) with ways of being and knowing. By doing this, we were calling on a rich tradition of looking to the ancestors, of birthing ourselves into a village and delivering each other into deeper communal scholarship. These are our stories, from educating preschoolers to high schoolers while building up our children as human beings.

As we individually and collectively parent our children, we are also caring for and nurturing our sisterhood as Black women scholars. We continue to care for ourselves by rejecting the white patriarchal notion of self-sacrifice. We reject the notion of a "do everything for others but ask nothing in return" mothering in favor of a sensibility of Black motherhood. We embrace a healthier sense of motherhood. We are growing independence, fostering community, and deconstructing secrets of working around systems meant to tear us down—these are distinctive traits of BLACK motherhood. These ideas are not new, as we cite other thinkers in this essay, but we have begun to think of them and this collective working of Black otherhood as a distinct type of epistemology. The intersection of Black womanhood, feminism, and motherhood creates its own means of praxis and support in knowledge production and nurturing of scholarship.

We begin with Candace's (Dace's) discussion of the roles of motherschooling versus homeschooling. Tehia then explores the rationale for modifying curriculum and discusses the methods used to expand her children's curriculum so they saw themselves in it, as a form of resistance and joy. Next, Kendra details the internal conflict we often feel as sisterscholars who engaged in motherscholarship by enrolling our children in the historically racist U.S. school system while simultaneously fighting for racial justice through intellectual discourse and activism. She discusses how this conflict was exacerbated during COVID-19, and how she leaned on her sensibilities of Black motherhood for resolve as a Black woman. Janaka gives a frame of community and scholarly engagement in mother- and sisterscholarship. Finally, Kaja shares the response of a family with small children to racial events during the pandemic. We end with a call for motherschooling advocacy in educational policy.

Dace

There were approximately 1.6 million children who were "homeschooled" in 2016, with 132,000 self-identifying as Black (Snyder, de Brey, and Dillow 2019). That number dramatically increased in March 2020 through "emergency" learning, when schools were shut down and kids were sent home. There is a distinct difference between planned homeschooling for a designated academic period of time and the abrupt shift in learning at home that occurred due to the global

COVID-19 pandemic. In addition to our professional positions, mothers in homes were expected to serve additional roles ranging from principal, teacher, and computer technician to custodian and "lunch lady." We call this "motherschooling," but this new educational territory also provided me a space to teach new—and review previously known—important skills and principles to my children.

I never received formal homeschooling as a child, but I was taught at home. I was a public education latchkey kid, with two working parents who instilled the principles of God, family, and education. My home education consisted of my parents talking about their educational experiences before and after the 1954 *Brown v. Board of Education* ruling. I got the "You gotta be twice as good" speech and my mother taught me that having an education was the one thing nobody could ever take from me (Hoff 2016). In agreement, my father also encouraged me to marry an educated man because he didn't want "stupid grandchildren" (he really did say that). They believed in being, as Cooper articulates it, "active school choice-makers and educational advocates" (2007, 508) before doing so was the norm.

As a mom of two teenage girls (sixteen and thirteen) and a teenage boy (fourteen), I have learned how to successfully advocate in their private educational learning spaces. Several of the advocacy moments that have seemed redundant as my children have moved from elementary to middle and now high school include challenging teachers to be more inclusive of the historical Black experience (and not just during Black History Month), speaking with administration about ways of recruiting a more diverse faculty and family representation, and reminding the school staff that students are learning directly from the example they set. These experiences have taught my children how to advocate for themselves, as they are more often than not one of few (if not the only) Black children in their classrooms. They have learned they will need to ask the difficult questions to their teachers and peers to further develop conversations and equally know that they do not have to nor can they speak for all Black people when asked for the "Black perspective."

I did not consider the question of equity in homeschooling and, in my naivete, thought my children's experience in private school would afford us a smoother transition into the collective homeschool process. I was wrong. While my eldest daughter and son were competent in their navigation of Zoom and Google, my youngest had not received any instruction with Google and we spent the first two weeks learning and advocating for her educational process. This consisted of us trying out new applications within the learning platforms, going to her siblings and asking for help, emailing the teachers (who were unable to assist us because they hadn't received online teaching training), and then literally high-fiving and jumping for joy when she submitted work successfully. They all learned that being a professor does not mean I "automagically" know everything about teaching.

Outside of formal instruction, being home gave our family time to talk collectively about the impact of COVID-19 on the Black community. As a public health faculty member, it was second nature for me to talk to my kids and increase their awareness of the disparities Black people face because of the choices made by those we vote into political offices and sometimes because of the behavioral choices we make. We discussed how this pandemic could either positively or negatively affect their own physical, mental, and spiritual health. They were open to my husband and I asking, "How are you feeling today?" and giving us honest, open answers instead of the usual teenage one-word, closed-ended response (e.g., "Fine").

As we moved into the summer, the formal online learning process ended with their school year, but the schooling did not. They learned the principles of business and the necessity of advocacy. We spoke to them about Black Wall Street and the importance of supporting Black businesses (Messer, Shriver, and Allison 2018). We tried to teach them skills of being business savvy through the game Monopoly, but after a little more than half a dozen games we had to stop playing because teenage attitudes were raggedy at The Man (husband's nickname), who kept winning the game (but had never played). (He is a smart guy, though. See? I listened to my parents.)

The social injustice unfolding across the country took us on a journey of delving even deeper into the subjects of racism and advocacy. During the summer, we took an in-depth look at the civil rights movement through our DVD collection of PBS's *Eyes on the Prize* (Pollard et al. 1987) so my children could see and hear the voices of those who charged change in our country. Those videos unexpectedly served as an introduction to their visceral feelings of racism being the "dumbest thing ever" (in their words). But they also served as an introduction to my children knowing they can make a difference even when their country is in a pandemic. After witnessing the needed continued advocacy for civil rights, following the murders of Black men and women previously mentioned, they learned to find ways to advocate safely. They took the opportunity to create and perform the online play *Mars Middle II: Emotional Space* (Justice Theater Project 2020), which had underlying tones of social justice, with other company kids from the Justice Theater Project. When Ahmaud Arbery was murdered, they agreed we should go for a 2.23-mile run/walk. It was the least they felt they could do, in that moment, to honor his life.

This is what motherschooling teenagers, while Black, looks like. It is supporting them in their "formal education" and combining that with the education they need from a Black perspective. It is dynamic, moving beyond the safety of our home. The pandemic forced many changes, including the realization of my legacy of raising active educational advocates. This educational legacy is alive with my grandmother, the first Black court reporter for the County of St. Louis, Missouri, to my mother, the first Black U.S. assistant district attorney for the Northern District of Iowa, to me—the first in our family to earn a doctor of philosophy. We did not get to those spaces in life without both formal and Black-perspective education and advocacy, and I can't wait to see where my children's collective education takes them!

Tehia

As the pandemic began, my preschool-age boys were now at home with my partner and me, and we both work full time. We asked ourselves how in the world we were going to make all of this work. We had to create some semblance of a schedule so we could be productive and ensure the boys' education didn't suffer. As a former elementary school teacher, and now an educational psychologist and teacher educator, I've been able to consistently use my teaching skills to empower whomever I was working with, from children to adults. I know the flaws in the education system: I've lived them, researched them, and work daily to dismantle the racism that exists. Back then, and even more so now, there was an opportunity here for me to affirm my children and be able to teach more of the Black history I knew was missing in their curriculum.

Racial socialization has always occurred in schools, through the curriculum and pedagogy, textbooks, teacher and administrative personnel, and policies and practices, among other things (Allen et al. 2017; Love 2019; Tatum 2017). White supremacy still exists in all of these spaces, in subtle and not so subtle ways of attempting to socialize Black children as inferior (Thomas and Speight 1999). Infrastructure and practices like whitewashed curriculum, behavioral norms that center whiteness and punish children that do not conform, the disregard of African American Vernacular English, and the unchecked bias of teachers have harmed Black children for centuries. With a research focus on culturally responsive teaching and anti-racism in schools, the need to disrupt the racism and bias that exists in teachers and students' perspectives has always been pertinent for me, even before I had children of my own. Now that I have children, I have volunteered and shared my expertise in the boys' preschool classrooms pre-pandemic to make sure that, at minimum, their curriculum had some anti-racist content when it came to holidays and history, and to remind teachers that being color blind is NOT okay. The reality is that I can't physically be in the school every day to advocate for what is needed to learn at school, so we supplemented at home. Motherschooling during and even prior to this pandemic was an opportunity to provide counter narratives of what school should look and feel like. What emerged was the curriculum that we—I, my husband, the boys, and my sisterscholars—revised and created!

The ways in which I saw my boys thrive while they were at home, despite COVID-19, spoke to how many Black boys experience school. At home, they were not under the shadow of biased teaching and curriculum (Delpit 2019; Gay 2014; Muhammad 2020). They were affirmed in the content we gave them as parents. We told them about who they are, the greatness of their ancestors, and how they survived through generations of trauma and became inventors, scientists, entrepreneurs, great scholars, literary geniuses, and everything else, via stories, documentaries, books, lessons, and websites. It was not too early to begin having these conversations about race, racism, and antiracism with preschoolers. We are not "afforded the privilege of [maintaining] innocence" (Goff et al. 2014, 539). Children are being racially socialized as young as three (Clark and Clark 1939), and we have to tell them who they are before the world tries to tell them who they are not. We ensured that their home library had books whose characters and authors look like and represent them, that the media they consumed had children who look like them—and for the shows that did not, we helped them critically question, Why aren't there any Brown or Black children on this show? From the paint and crayons that match their skin tone to the activity webinars we selected, the boys saw themselves in what they were doing or learning. This was and is crucial as they pay attention to what they see, what we say, and how we behave.

My husband and I modeled for the boys the excellence of Blackness (we define excellence as the diverse range of Black folx doing average and awesome things in the face of oppression), as well as being as silly as possible so they can experience sheer joy every day! I repurposed and customized resources from the college courses I teach on education, brainstormed with my sisterscholars, and enrolled in monthly subscriptions of Black history content, just to name a few things. The options for showing them what Black excellence looks like were limitless. In June, Black Music Month, I used my Black history subscription service to center Black music artists such as Prince, Duke Ellington, Miles Davis, and Nina Simone (among many others). We watched old videos of those musicians performing and connected them to math, language arts, social studies, and geography, all within the context of Blackness and Black history. For Juneteenth, we colored Juneteenth flags (shared with the other motherschoolers), took a virtual field trip to Rochester, NY, to learn more about Frederick Douglass, danced in a virtual drum circle, and participated in a drive-by Juneteenth parade. It warmed our hearts that the boys experienced so much joy that day. It was also exhausting having to comb through so much content, then build lessons and activities around what I found, as I still navigate COVID-19, work, and household duties. In the end, it was worth it, because my boys and the other motherschooled children got to see themselves in the content they were learning. If not for my sisterscholars, the spring, summer, and fall of 2020 would've been a far more difficult experience for both the adults and children in my household. Motherschooling provided me the space to be creative as a form of resistance and to affirm and center my Black children through the curriculum we designed as a community.

Kendra

The year 2020 took us for a loop, didn't it? In January, we were all excited and visionary. Remember all those "20/20 vision" sermons, memes, and vision boards? I, too, was excited about 2020. I planned to get married in April and honeymoon in Jamaica. My daughter would start middle school, and we had a family trip to the Caribbean planned for Christmas break. As a tenure-track assistant professor, my promotion and tenure packet was due in the fall. Personally, and professionally, I had been waiting for this time my whole life—the time when everything was finally coming together.

By February, however, the unexpected death of basketball great Kobe Bryant and the relentless Australian forest fires shocked the world. These tragedies were destined to be "the" events of 2020. By spring, hardly anyone recalled the fires. We were, instead, consumed by the effects of COVID-19. Then, the world as we knew it stopped. Well, for us, the world did not actually stop; it went online. Immediately, as a single and full-time working parent, I was thrust into helping my eleven-year-old daughter transition into remote learning while I transitioned my college courses online. We sheltered in place, only leaving the house for groceries. For a few weeks, life was precarious and nerve racking. Then we created a routine. We focused all our energy on healthier eating, completing school and work assignments, and exercising to reduce stress. That was it: to not allow the pandemic to consume our sanity and to resist it by strengthening our immune system. Managing the chaos became the norm, yet, like an episode of *The Twilight Zone*, time moved in slow motion, leaving much time for self-reflection and resulting in inspiration and resolve. I'll start with my thoughts on my daughter's education.

As a sociologist with expertise in racial inequality, I have always seriously side-eyed the education system for pushing a white, heteronormative educational agenda (Ferfolja 2007; Crichlow 2013) where "white is right" and non-white and non-cisgender contributions are misrepresented, minimized, or ignored. Just as mine was, my daughter's public education is centered in whiteness: white history, white economics, white social studies, white language arts. I have always been a critic of the white supremacist public education experience of the United States, which is especially detrimental in schools like my daughter attends, which is 97 percent students of color. However, her school was a magnet school, with recognition for academic excellence, much like the magnet school education I had myself. As a "successful" product of the magnet school system, I enrolled my daughter with the intention of correcting, clarifying, and supplementing her white-centric education with Black knowledge, Black history, and cultural appreciation. We watch Black films and relate it to class content; we pick Black historical figures and events to do projects and reports on (when given freedom to choose); we read books with Black characters, authors, and representation for class assignments. We center African history in her homework, such as when she did a second grade "My Family's Immigration Story" assignment and traced her heritage back to our unknown roots in Africa. Even though my family has been able to trace our ancestry to a plantation in South Carolina, we pushed the narrative in this lesson across the Atlantic to acknowledge and honor our unknown-to-us ancestors.

I was okay with this arrangement until I overheard my daughter's Black fifth-grade teacher during her online language arts class during COVID-19. In an exchange with a ten-year-old Black boy, the teacher asked, "What would your life be like if you took on the role of the [book] character and were alive in the mid-1800s?" He answered, "If I was alive back then, I would most likely be a slave." She quipped, "That's not right," and moved on to another student. She dismissed him. He grumbled under his breath, which I took as an indication that he felt dismissed. As an educator, I understood the teacher was trying to keep the lesson on track and focus on identifying text evidence in literature, but as a Black parent, I was enraged. A young Black boy, who was critically thinking about a historical context and creative arts question, was made invisible by his Black teacher and this was witnessed by his peers. He should have been celebrated. I cannot speak of the teacher's intention. This small window into her world

illuminated the racial microaggressions and Eurocentric domination built into the curriculum (Johnston-Goodstar and VeLue Roholt
2017) that non-white students experience, and it led me to more fully
question my role and responsibility in my daughter's learning. In an
effort to counter these experiences, I enrolled my daughter in Passport to Cultural Freedom, a supplementary six-week online course
offered through the nonprofit, Black woman–owned organization
Jelani Gives, where girls aged eleven to fifteen explore and rediscover
Black history through the lens of Africa. The organization's founder,
Ashley N. Company, created the program to "unlearn false narratives
taught through the U.S. education system and grow their sense of
pride and cultural identity" (Jelani Gives n.d.).

I then turned to my sisterscholars and we began engaging in thoughtful conversations about our similar situations. We shared stories, some
quite unbelievable, like when Kaja shared that a teacher called her
mixed-race son a "mutt," or when my daughter's teacher issued a three-
day-late rule on assignments with "NO EXCEPTIONS" during a pandemic when so many children lacked internet, computers, sanity, and
stable homes to complete assignments on time. We questioned how
we, as Black women mothers and scholars, are in a complicated and
dynamic relationship with white supremacy, as outsiders-within (Collins 1998). Black feminist theorist Patricia Hill Collins (1998) argues
that Black women, although structurally oppressed, have historically
confronted economic and social injustice. We are now positioned as the
liaisons between the white and Black community. As academicians, we
have learned how to successfully navigate in a white world, and we can
talk about racial injustice to white and Black folk comfortably.

As a Black woman of the academy, I am in a newly experienced
and privileged position of having educational and technical knowledge, social support, and financial stability for my immediate family,
which my child directly benefits from. However, these privileges do
not protect me from the guilt I feel that close family and friends, and

many others in the Black community, are suffering when it comes to health, education access, and employment. I also gave up the division between my home and work life that often enables my ability to be productive at work and supermom when I'm at home. And COVID-19 exposed another quandary: Do I put more time into being a thought leader, social justice activist, and community leader when it comes to addressing the injustices exposed by COVID-19 and related killings of Black men, women, and children by the police? Or should I put more energy into affirming Black education for my daughter at home? Either way, in the context of COVID-19, each task seemed exhausting. Would I be voluntarily adding to the exhaustion I experience as a Black woman? As a mother? As a teacher? As a Black woman motherschooling? As a sister, daughter, aunt, granddaughter, friend, and wife?

That is when I leaned into my understanding of motherschooling, where I have community as a Black woman. I am not alone, and I grant myself grace in a system that was designed for Black women to be laborers by contributing only to the benefit of other systems and populations (Rousseau 2013), a system that was never our own. I resist this social construction of expectations over my life. I have succeeded in preserving my child's joy, as she is thriving at home. I have centered and protected her Blackness and uplifted my Black male husband. I have fought for her liberation from a white-centric education and my own liberation by not putting on a cape and figuring out "racism" for my white colleagues on demand, even as I am under evaluation for tenure and promotion. But I have also been myself. I can do many things well, but it is not my responsibility to be everything for everyone. Some things will slip through the cracks and fall to the wayside (e.g., housework, homework, coursework), and that is okay. As long as my family is healthy, safe, and secure, we will be all right. At times, I take on too much anyway. However, I will fight for my existence and the existence and fair treatment of those I love, and I love my community.

Janaka

In early March 2020, I was between two conferences during our campus's spring break. One was a daylong meeting for the National Women's Studies Association program department chairs and directors, plus an overnight, that I am excited to attend every year. The conversation on how to adapt our programs and thrive in the face of state restrictions in states that don't overwhelmingly support women's, gender, and sexuality studies, was fruitful. Presentations included topics such as overcoming difficulties in getting tenure despite stringent academic and service contributions and keeping curriculum vibrant with limited funding.

I returned home to one sick child (strep throat), who returned to school for a couple days as I prepared for a Black women's leadership conference in another state—the same day another one of my children came home with a fever. I took her to the doctor—not strep. She went to school the day I planned to leave and was sick again. We went back to the doctor, and she was diagnosed with the flu (even with the vaccine). My spouse also works on campus and took the next day off, and I drove that evening to attend this much anticipated gathering of "my" people. After the opening session of the conference that Friday morning, everyone was sent home because of COVID-19 (and believe me, I checked for cancellations before driving). Months later, and this was still where we were except for deciding whether to send our children back to school one day a week or go completely virtual, with an additional extension before our academic campus planned to go back mostly in person, although with hybrid and online options.

"This is crazy," I heard myself saying again and again among my friend and colleague groups. Many of us are working mothers with also working spouses or partners. Mine also finished his doctoral degree while working full time during the first phase of shutdown. Meetings and work obligations continued, all while sheltering in place.

Even events that had taken place sporadically ramped up once people discovered the magic of Zoom, and then it became a dance between wanting to be present, protecting my family's privacy, and having other needs to meet.

To be clear here, my children were not the problem. When people say things such as "It must be so hard to be a parent," I also feel the need to assert that I enjoy the choice I made to have a family even while acknowledging that I also don't believe it's for everyone. The problem was that many people used the opportunity of knowing where I was—as an employee, administrator, scholar, and parent—to rewrite their needs and, literally, to be seen.[2]

Even with the stress of the pandemic and added racialized trauma that continued in our society, I enjoyed the time I was able to recommit to my children—to knowing what they were learning and wanted to learn, to evaluating firsthand what they were doing in school—which I otherwise would not have. As the conditions of COVID-19 continued with loss in close and distant circles and the tragedies of Black women, men, and nonbinary folx unfolded on our screens and in our timelines, not to mention those deaths that would go unmentioned, I was deeply saddened at the additional education that I was then led to provide my children on histories of anti-Blackness in America.

With my work as a professor of African American literature, talking about why Black people were being killed by police and why they were showing it on television was not the conversation I wanted to have with then six- and nine-year-old little Black girls and a young Black boy, and yet they were necessary. As the world told them their lives didn't matter, I had to reiterate that they had always mattered.

In come principles of motherschooling, the informal community system of education that we have relied on since I have been a professional Black mother. As an assistant professor at a larger state university with predominantly older faculty members in my unit, I can't honestly say that there was an overwhelmingly large support system in my department. People were nice and excited, but there was either a notion of forgetting what having a family felt like in a new position (or any position at all, for that matter), or a curiosity as to whether one could be a serious academic with children, whatever that means. In "The Metaphysical Dilemma: Academic Black Women," Janelle L. Williams and Ayana Hardaway discuss the multiple roles that Black women academics hold, from daughter, to sister, to wife and mother, while "Academic, researcher, doctor, professor, scholar [are] titles typically attributed to men" (2018, 113). Yet we value these roles in addition to our relationships with each other. We also acknowledge our needs for support of a village, which has been discussed by scholars and activists such as Angela Davis in "Reflections on the Black Woman's Role in the Community of Slaves," where she argues of the Black matriarch, "her concern and struggles for physical survival, while clearly important, did not constitute her most outstanding contributions . . . by virtue of the brutal force of circumstances, the black woman was assigned the mission of promoting the consciousness of resistance" (1971, 113).

Fortunately, I had groups of Black women and multiracial families going through the same things at the same time. In my children's younger years, I had Mocha Moms, a national Black women's organization that supported me through the early years with playdates, mom's nights out, and thinking through issues of physical and emotional health for our families. And at work, I had an informal network of colleagues and sister-mothers called Sister Educators Eating Dinner(s) — which I named and nicknamed "SEEDS" — with whom I ate, discussed challenges and celebrated successes in academia, and collaborated on just what we would do with kids at different stages (the kids also became great friends).

When "the 'Rona" brought us home in March 2020, I depended on these colleagues for continued support through virtual writing groups, wine nights, and sisterly chat. Our kids found solace in making sense of what was going on in the world too. We could not do It alone and fortunately didn't have to. When I took to writing five responses in as many weeks on the relationships between the pandemic and anti-Black violence (and how white friends and colleagues seemed to see the challenges as strictly related to their educational access vis-à-vis COVID) (Lewis 2020a, 2020b), these communities were also my support systems, spaces where we could all share tips and conversations within our fields and even just send pictures of childhood joy (which I also continue to appreciate).

Likewise, when the end of the school year became difficult due to my children's natural exhaustion from the ongoing time in front of the screen without the context of seeing "why" assignments were important, I was able to help shape the relevance to us. My son was dejected when an essay about abolitionist figures (including Sojourner Truth) was sent back for being too long (they were asked to write a one- to two-sentence summary). On the other hand, he was excited to read in a class assignment about freedom fighters. We had him keep the full essay (five paragraphs) and add the "abstract" on top of it. Family schooling, check. Fourth-grade assignment on monuments in North Carolina? He worked on it while I wrote with the sisterscholars, and one sisterscholar challenged him with these questions: "What monuments exist to Black community figures and histories? Where are they? Who built them?" He did his research and I learned that day too.

I am not my kids' primary educator, even as they have returned to remote learning in the fall, but I am an educator both to them and to my own students. But most importantly, at least from my perspective when the primary figure(s) in the home are also working, I am modeling what a Black mother and educator is. We selected opportunities for them to learn from people who look like them (Black women educators and histories through Outschool and a summer reading program through a local Black educator). We are working as a family with other families to launch a business that matches local educators, educational services, nonprofits, and students to maximize learning opportunities. Based on our fields of knowledge, we collaborate on tools and topics to optimize community success. Ultimately, we supplement but also shift their understanding of what and how to learn their history and culture and how social events affect us specifically even as they are framed broadly within the mainstream. With and beyond COVID-19, motherschooling and family support allows our children to understand that yes, their Black lives and Black love matter.

Kaja

I live in the busy. My life is brimming with a house full of boys, ages three, six, and ten. Until recently I was the only Black professor in my department; I work in a largely white field (theatre) (Pierce 2020). As an acting teacher and practitioner, I don't have the predictability of a writing schedule, as auditions and speaking engagements sometimes give little notice. I live in spaces not created for mothers or Black women. I find myself as the "other" that Collins defines in her work. In *Black Feminist Thought*, Collins suggests that the Black woman is the outsider, the stranger, the one who doesn't belong, whom society uses as a boundary to define who does. The notion of the Black woman as the other "provides ideological justification for race, gender, and class oppression" (Collins 1990, 69–70). Being an outsider means traversing and navigating spaces for the survival of ourselves and our children, a process we are calling motherschooling.

We employed this practice of motherschooling as we isolated, as we negotiated a disrupted, unprepared public education system, as we affirmed Black Lives Matter. Angela Davis notes in "Reflections on the Black Woman's Role in the Community of Slaves," "The black woman in chains could help to lay the foundation for some degree of autonomy, both for herself and her men. Even as she was suffering under her unique oppression as female, she was thrust by the force of circumstances into the center of the slave community. She was, therefore, essential to the survival of the community. Not all people have survived enslavement; hence her survival-oriented activities were themselves a form of resistance" (1971, 7). As a mother, "survival" meant countering harmful remarks overheard on Zoom by teachers about protestors and a narrow history curriculum by researching the roots of my maternal side's Cape Verdean liberation narrative. I assigned one of my sons a report over the summer on his great-great-uncle who fought alongside Amílcar Cabral. Suddenly his Wakanda-themed room had real African hero posters on the wall. When he finished his report, he came to me and said, "We come from a family of freedom fighters. I need to make sure I make a difference." I read about the plight of Black communities while I and other Black mothers did what we have always done: embrace our children, make four cents out of two, and figure out the impossible. While this navigation was hard, there was opportunity to shape and protect my children in a moment of widespread trauma.

In comparison, while the *New York Times* ran headlines from white parents like "'I Have Given Up': Parenting in Quarantine" and "I Refuse to Run a Coronavirus Home School" (Harris and Tarchak 2020; Weiner 2020), we glanced at this, empathized, and then rolled up our sleeves. For us, quitting wasn't an option. Our children were not going to be okay in an educational system set up for their failure. Within the first three weeks of the school shutdown, my sisterscholars and I were trading Afrocentric homeschool curricula and Google spreadsheets of free educational resources, sharing what we'd learned about free afterschool programs with information about food and aid, donating and organizing supplies, and exchanging information about the spread of and protection from COVID. In 2020, we were doing the work described by Davis and the work that later generations of Black women had done—for example, the women of the Black Panther Party, especially in Oakland, where the system was set up for women to be "mothers and revolutionaries," as they "adopted collective parenting, caring for one another's children as they carried out their . . . tasks" (Williams 2013, 119). Instinctually, we were mirroring our foremothers.

In the language of Roby and Cook, my fellow motherschoolers and I, "through intentional and collaborative duo-ethnographic work, have come together to grow as Black feminist scholars; *it is through these acts of love that we purposefully sought opportunities to work together and support one another in difficult and challenging anti-Black spaces*" (2019, 6; emphasis mine). Those anti-Black spaces could include our workplaces, our children's schools, and the country we were living in. Yet we worked together to create spaces of joy. Motherschooling gave us a measure of inoculation against the stress, worry, and panic of our writing period by giving us a community and a sounding board. It gave us encouragement and laughter and a place to exist and work without judgment as we learned and thought about how to shelter and teach our children.

In one instance, we donned regalia, invited family, and set up a full Zoom commencement, complete with the Black national anthem and certificates of achievement for every child, to substitute for missed promotion and advancement celebrations. We had the children in caps and gowns, and each mother took a section of the program. At other times, I set up camp themes like dinosaur week, space week, and Zoom script readings. This was done not for social media glory, but as acts of liberation to preserve our children's peace and childhood as things fell apart around them.

In the chaos of all we were encountering, I had to remember that the ability to experience joy and celebration amid brutal pain is also part of the Black woman's inheritance. So I consoled my frightened three-year-old when a sheriff's car led the teacher parade through our neighborhood a week after the police brutally murdered George

Floyd; he asked if they were going to hurt us. After I comforted him, we snuggled and made dinosaur soap. We watched the KidLit4Black-Lives Rally (2020) on YouTube and then built a tire swing. I dealt with fumbled solidarity statements at work and then we planted a beautiful garden (which I privately referred to as my rage garden). I had a meeting with my oldest child's principal over the use of the N-word in class and a teacher referring to my child as a "mutt," and then we made pizza. In the first terrifying days of the pandemic, we turned giant boxes into "cars" using leftover paint, parked them in the living room, and did a drive-in movie night. Not because my heart wasn't breaking, but because none of this was new to us.

I was nine when my stepfather was brutally pulled from his car and searched and harassed by police during the Charles Stuart attacks in Boston.[3] I remember the trauma and fear I experienced while waiting for him to come home and then wondering why he couldn't go back to work for a week. I experienced all of this as the police smashed and ruined Black neighborhoods. So yes, none of this is new, and navigating the spaces that my children were now experiencing compounded my own memories as well.

Full Reflection and Forward Movement

We entered into this writing space in spring of 2020 full of frustration and despair, but equally full of hope and promise. Our first few months of collaboration were not of writing but sharing ideas, stories, and strategies from each of our varied lives. Based on our individual and collective experiences, we came together to argue that Black mothers are educators and should be at the table when decisions are being made concerning education, family, and policy. Our voices are critical and central, as we have navigated this terrain for decades. We hope this essay inspires others, as it has for us, to advocate for Black children and demand educational policy changes at all levels, to use our experiences to shape curriculum pushing cultural competence and anti-racism and to eliminate microaggression and punitive pipelines.

Our greatest hope is that the effects of COVID-19 will wane and our children will resume their formally known in-person communities. And yet our role as motherschoolers is to ensure they return to that world more aware of who they are as Black people and of what, in relation to Blackness, is being ignored in the classroom. Davis's work on Black women in community reminds us that even in struggle, brutality, and pain, we all have choices about *if* our children will return to the education system or if we will create new and exciting spaces of learning in our homes and communities. We have come to understand that motherschooling is not secondary but essential to learning. We have chosen to give our children space to determine *how* they will return to the education system. They are poised to advocate for themselves, speak of Black excellence, successfully navigate in a white world, create new and exciting spaces of learning in their communities, and ultimately know that their Black lives and our Black love matter because of their experiences at home. Like our motherschooling, their supplemented knowledge is not secondary to what is learned in the classroom but essential to and in conjunction with their classroom learning. Lastly, our children also know that we will continue to advocate for their needs to disrupt academic harm.

Conclusion

Motherschooling is communal. It is sometimes dependent on others to fill in gaps and offer encouragement. Motherschooling principles allow us to be frustrated with the decisions made for our children that do not consider varied learning styles, access, and the ability of Black children. When these situations arise, we quickly debate what works best for our working families, while being fully aware that all children don't have the access or previous experience to do independent work. Motherschooling allows our Black children to navigate fear and anxiety. It prepares them for how the world may treat them and gives context to what they see on the morning news. It allows Black children to build healthy relationships with others. It nurtures Black boys and girls as they are, on their own terms.

Motherschooling also affirms that we do the best we can for our children, and we don't sacrifice their education for the world's convenience. We return focus to them that has been taken away and given to things that are not as important. We also realize that we are called to be othermothers (Collins 1990) in the schooling process—as we have continued responsibilities to each other and to villages of children outside our neighborhoods. Motherschooling contends that we are also responsible for Black families and children, and we are all connected through policy and practice. We create structures for our children to learn at their best (well fed, well loved, and seen) and to unlearn those practices that don't speak to them being their best selves (strict focus on behavior rather than what is behind misbehavior). We set values on their lives and the livelihood of our family to negotiate a balance for our home in which needs are centered collectively. We make kinship and community the structure that replaces punitive measures as we center our individual and collective needs.

This multi-ethnographic approach reinforces key principles of motherschooling—valuing and empowering our child(ren). We value each other (as motherscholars and sisterscholars) as we value our families and our communities. We see that we must *all* be well to not just survive but thrive. We experience our lives both separately and in community because we acknowledge the power in our individuality, uniqueness, and togetherness. As we advocate for ourselves, we model advocacy for our children as the next generation of change agents and sustainers of our collective soul.

Notes

1. This was Executive Order No. 118 Limiting Operations of Restaurants and Bars and Broadening Unemployment Insurance Benefits in Response to COVID-19; the full text can be accessed at https://files.nc.gov/governor/documents/files/EO118.pdf.

2. I discuss the needs of Black women, and specifically mothers, in the academy in "Brown Girls in the Ivory Tower" (Lewis 2017).

3. On October 23, 1989 Charles Stuart, a wealthy banker, shot and killed his pregnant wife in Boston and shot himself in the stomach. He told police and the community that a Black man did it. He was a domestic abuser and was angry that his wife refused to get an abortion. For thirteen minutes while she tried to survive, he refused to assist the police so that they could locate her. What followed were days of terror by the police department, ordered by then mayor Ray Flynn, who ordered an all-out assault, sending every available officer to the Mission Hill housing project, a mostly Black area, and also terrorizing Black men driving in and out of Boston for work, like my stepfather. Mayor Flynn said at the time, "I demand that the Boston Police Department continue to be extremely aggressive in cracking down on people who are using guns to kill innocent people. . . . It's intolerable. We will use every lawful tool to support our police officers in cracking down on gun-wielding criminals" (Scalese 2014).

Bibliography

Allen, Ayana, Stephen D. Hancock, Tehia Starker-Glass, and Chance W. Lewis. 2017. "Mapping Culturally Relevant Pedagogy into Teacher Education Programs: A Critical Framework." *Teachers College Record* 119, no. 1 (January): 1–26. https://doi.org/10.1177%2F016146811711900107.

Berry, Daina Ramey, and Kali Nicole Gross. 2020. *A Black Women's History of the United States*. ReVisioning American History, vol. 5. Boston: Beacon Press.

Clark, Kenneth B., and Mamie K. Clark. 1939. "The Development of Consciousness of Self and the Emergence of Racial Identification in Negro Preschool Children." *Journal of Social Psychology* 10, no. 4: 591–99. https://psycnet.apa.org/doi/10.1080/00224545.1939.9713394.

Collins, Patricia Hill. 1990. *Black Feminist Thought: Knowledge, Consciousness, and the Politics of Empowerment*. New York: Routledge.

———. 1998. *Fighting Words: Black Women and the Search for Justice*. Contradictions Series, vol. 7. Minneapolis: University of Minnesota Press.

Cooper, Anna Julia. *A Voice from the South.* (1892) 1988. Xenia, OH: Aldine Printing House. Reprint, New York: Oxford University Press. Citations refer to the Oxford University Press edition.

Cooper, Camille Wilson. 2007. "School Choice as 'Motherwork': Valuing African-American Women's Educational Advocacy and Resistance." *International Journal of Qualitative Studies in Education* 20, no. 5 (August): 491–512. https://doi.org/10.1080/09518390601176655.

Crichlow, Warren. 2013. *Race, Identity, and Representation in Education.* New York: Routledge.

Davis, Angela. 1971. "Reflections on the Black Woman's Role in the Community of Slaves." *Black Scholar* 3, no. 4 (December): 2–15. https://doi.org/10.1080 /00064246.1971.11431201.

Delpit, Lisa. 2019. *Teaching When the World Is on Fire.* New York: New Press.

Ferfolja, Tania. 2007. "Schooling Cultures: Institutionalizing Heteronormativity and Heterosexism." *International Journal of Inclusive Education* 11, no. 2 (February): 147–62. https://doi.org/10.1080/13603110500296596.

Gay, Geneva. 2014. "Culturally Responsive Teaching Principles, Practices, and Effects." In *Handbook of Urban Education,* edited by Richard H. Milner and Kofi Lomotey, 353–72. New York: Routledge.

Goff, Phillip Atiba, Matthew Christian Jackson, Brooke Allison Lewis Di Leone, Carmen Marie Culotta, and Natalie Ann DiTomasso. 2014. "The Essence of Innocence: Consequences of Dehumanizing Black Children." *Journal of Personality and Social Psychology* 106, no. 4: 526–45. https://psycnet.apa.org /doi/10.1037/a0035663.

Harris, Rachel L., and Lisa Tarchak. 2020. "'I Have Given Up': Parenting in Quarantine." *New York Times,* May 13, 2020. https://www.nytimes.com/2020 /05/13/opinion/parenting-coronavirus-burnout.html.

Hoff, Pamela Twyman. 2016. "'Fool Me Once, Shame on You; Fool Me Twice, Shame on Me': African American Students' Reclamation of Smartness as Resistance." *Race, Ethnicity, and Education* 19, no. 6 (April): 1200–1208. https:// doi.org/10.1080/13613324.2016.1168542.

hooks, bell. *Teaching to Transgress.* 1994. New York: Routledge.

Jelani Gives. n.d. "Passport to Cultural Freedom." Accessed July 2, 2022. https:// crownedbyjelani.com/products/passport-to-cultural-freedom?_pos=1and _sid=99ced7ba2and_ss=r.

Johnston-Goodstar, Katie, and Ross VeLure Roholt. 2017. "'Our Kids Aren't Dropping Out; They're Being Pushed Out': Native American Students and Racial Microaggressions in Schools." *Journal of Ethnic and Cultural Diversity in Social Work* 26, no. 1–2 (February): 30–47. https://doi.org/10.1080/1531 3204.2016.1263818.

Justice Theater Project. 2020. *Mars Middle II: Emotional Space.* Streamed August 1, 2020. YouTube video, 1:02:21. https://www.youtube.com/watch?v= mUHoFQL9kCs.

"KidLit4BlackLives Rally." 2020. Led by Kwame Alexander, Jacqueline Woodson, and Jason Reynolds. Brown Bookshelf. Streamed June 5, 2020. YouTube video, 2:14:41. https://www.youtube.com/watch?v=fElXu_MdRrs.

Lewis, Janaka B. 2017. "Brown Girls in the Ivory Tower: Reflections on Race, Gender, and Coming of Age in Academia." In *Coping with Gender Inequities: Critical Conversations of Women Faculty*, edited by Sherwood Thompson and Pam Parry, 159–70. Lanham, MD: Rowman and Littlefield.

———. 2020a. "On Behalf of My Sisters: A Self-Help Curriculum for White Women." Medium, May 30, 2020. https://janakabowman.medium.com/on -behalf-of-my-sisters-a-self-help-curriculum-for-white-women-ac42c72824e1.

———. 2020b. "Whose Bloody Hands? On Sanitizing American Experiences." Medium, June 7, 2020. https://janakabowman.medium.com/whose-bloody -hands-on-sanitizing-american-experiences-f04957993bd8.

Love, Bettina L. 2019. *We Want to Do More Than Survive: Abolitionist Teaching and the Pursuit of Educational Freedom.* Boston: Beacon Press.

Lynn, Marvin. 1999. "Toward a Critical Race Pedagogy: A Research Note." *Urban Education* 33, no. 5 (January): 606–26. https://doi.org/10.1177%2F00 42085999335004.

Martin, Jennifer L. 2014. "Critical Race Theory, Hip Hop, and Huck Finn: Narrative Inquiry in a High School English Classroom." *Urban Review* 46, no. 2 (June): 244–67. https://doi.org/10.1007/s11256-013-0250-9.

Matias, Cheryl E. 2016. "'Mommy, Is Being Brown Bad?' Critical Race Parenting in a Post-Race Era." *Race and Pedagogy Journal: Teaching and Learning for Justice* 1, no. 3: article 1. https://soundideas.pugetsound.edu/rpj/vol1 /iss3/1.

Messer, Chris M., Thomas E. Shriver, and Alison E Adams. 2018. "The Destruction of Black Wall Street: Tulsa's 1921 Riot and the Eradication of Accumulated Wealth." *American Journal of Economics and Sociology* 77, no. 3–4 (October): 789–819. https://doi.org/10.1111/ajes.12225.

Muhammad, Gholdy. 2020. *Cultivating Genius: An Equity Framework for Culturally and Historically Responsive Literacy.* New York: Scholastic.

Owens, Tammy. 2019. "Afterword: BlackGirlMagic Is Real." In *Black Girl Magic Beyond the Hashtag: Twenty-First-Century Acts of Self-Definition*, edited by

Julia Jordan-Zachery and Duchess Harris, 184–86. Tucson: University of Arizona Press.

Pierce, J. R. 2020. "'I Want to be Part of That': The Urgent Work of Diversifying White Theatre Staffs." *American Theatre*, August 6, 2020. https://www.americantheatre.org/2020/08/06/i-want-to-be-part-of-that-the-urgent-work-of-diversifying-white-theatre-staffs/.

Pollard, Samuel D., Sheila Curran Bernard, James A. DeVinney, and Madison Davis Lacy. 1987. *Eyes on the Prize*. Boston: Blackside Productions. DVD.

Roby, Reanna S., and Elizabeth B. Cook. 2019. "Black Women's Sharing in Resistance Within the Academy." *Taboo: The Journal of Culture and Education* 18, no. 1 (September): 5–17. https://doi.org/10.31390/taboo.18.1.02.

Rousseau, Nicole. 2013. "Historical Womanist Theory: Re-visioning Black Feminist Thought." *Race, Gender and Class*: 191–204. https://www.jstor.org/stable/43496941.

Scalese, Roberto. 2014. "The Charles Stuart Murders and the Racist Branding Boston Just Can't Seem to Shake." *Boston Globe*, October 22, 2014. https://www.boston.com/news/local-news/2014/10/22/the-charles-stuart-murders-and-the-racist-branding-boston-just-cant-seem-to-shake.

Snyder, Thomas D., Cristobal de Brey, and Sally A. Dillow. 2019. *Digest of Education Statistics 2017*. Washington, D.C.: National Center for Education Statistics. https://nces.ed.gov/pubs2018/2018070.pdf.

Tatum, Beverly Daniel. 2017. *Why Are All the Black Kids Sitting Together in the Cafeteria? And Other Conversations About Race*. New York: Basic Books.

Thomas, Anita Jones, and Suzette L. Speight. 1999. "Racial Identity and Racial Socialization Attitudes of African American Parents." *Journal of Black Psychology* 25, no. 2 (May): 152–70. https://doi.org/10.1177%2F0095798499025002002.

Weiner, Jennie. 2020. "I Refuse to Run a Coronavirus Home School." *New York Times*, March 19, 2020. https://www.nytimes.com/2020/03/19/opinion/coronavirus-home-school.html.

Williams, Jakobi. 2013. *From the Bullet to the Ballot: The Illinois Chapter of the Black Panther Party and Racial Coalition Politics in Chicago*. Chapel Hill: University of North Carolina Press.

Williams, Janelle L., and Ayana Tyler Hardaway. 2018. "The Metaphysical Dilemma: Academic Black Women." *Diverse: Issues in Higher Education*, September 20, 2018. https://diverseeducation.com/article/127139/.

CHAPTER 8

The Narratives of Black Women Techies

An In-Depth Qualitative Investigation of the Experiences of Black Women in Tech Organizations During the COVID-19 Pandemic

Breauna Marie Spencer

Introduction

Overall, the COVID-19 pandemic has brought about significant and disruptive changes across the globe, which include record unemployment rates. In May 2020, TrustRadius published the 2020 *Women in Tech Report*, which demonstrated the impact of COVID-19 on women in tech industries, concluding that women struggle to maintain a balance between work and personal life, fear employment insecurity and wage reduction, worry about how marginalized communities are being impacted by the pandemic, and must contend with other workplace stressors that could continue to adversely impact them socially, psychologically, and economically (Huisache 2020). To make matters worse, women in the tech sector were more likely to be laid off or furloughed than their male counterparts during the early part of the pandemic (Huisache 2020). Black women working in tech fields (e.g., academia and industry) experience a variety of social inequalities, ranging from systemic racism and sexism to exclusionism (Alegria 2020; Erete, Rankin, and Thomas 2020; Rankin and Thomas 2020; Thomas et al. 2018). Although many of these particular issues impact women of color more generally in tech, researchers know very little about the implications of the pandemic on Black women working in the tech field. Accordingly, it is imperative to examine Black women's experiences in tech organizations; this demographic population remains one of the most underrepresented groups in tech careers, both historically and contemporarily, due to systemic racism and sexism.

Black women's low numbers in tech careers could potentially become further exacerbated due to the pandemic. In addition, tech companies and firms have suffered major job losses, which I surmise may disproportionately affect Black women and other underrepresented groups (Condon 2020). To explore the lived experiences of Black women professionals in tech organizations during the pandemic, I conducted qualitative interviews with six Black women, guided by the following research question: What are the workplace experiences of Black female tech professionals prior to and during COVID-19? The research study utilizes discourse analysis to investigate Black women tech professionals' workplace experiences across race and gender, and the degree to which the pandemic has been a major catalyst for organizational change, either positively or negatively.

Black Women's Race-Gender Workplace Experiences

Historically, the experiences of Black women in the workplace have been and continue to be psychologically exhausting and taxing due to the intersection of their gender and race (Donovan et al. 2012; Hall, Everett, and Hamilton-Mason 2012). Black women are often the recipients of unfavorable stereotypes, including that they are angry, aggressive, strong, salacious, and caregiving matriarchs (Reynolds-Dobbs, Thomas, and Harrison 2008). These stereotypical depictions marginalize and oppress Black women in the workplace because "their credibility, authority, and skills are always questioned" (Reynolds-Dobbs,

Thomas, and Harrison 2008, 140). Black women also struggle incessantly to advance in their careers due to the effects of racism, sexism, and a lack of mentorship (Hague and Okpala 2017; Iheduru-Anderson 2020). Due to their experiences in the workplace, Black women also report a lack of sense of belonging and have become rather silent about the discrimination they encounter because they are "psychologically paralyzed"; they are mentally checked out due to their stressful social interactions and conversations with their non-Black colleagues, which is rooted in racism (Dickens and Chavez 2018, 766).

Black women also report having to negotiate their social identities at the intersection of their gender and race in the workplace as they are required to conceal parts of themselves or alter their behavior in order to fit into their organizational environments (Atewologun, Sealy, and Vinnicombe 2015; Dickens, Jones, and Hall 2020; Hall, Everett, and Hamilton-Mason 2012). This is because organizations were historically crafted and designed to uphold the "ideological, institutional, and physical norms that privilege Whiteness" as the established standard for all employees to abide by or follow (Wingfield and Alston 2014, 283). As such, Black women attempt to navigate working in predominately white organizations where they are often the lone Black woman, thus causing them to alter their social identities (Dickens, Womack, and Dimes 2019). Such responses can lead to race-related stress and identity issues (Gamst et al. 2020). Black women are also often misunderstood by their non-Black colleagues. This continuous state of being misunderstood comes with a host of social-psychological challenges, including stress, depression, and social isolation and alienation.

Jones and Shorter-Gooden explain how Black women's social identities are constantly misunderstood, misconstrued, and deemed inappropriate: "Indeed, because Black women exist against a backdrop of myth and stereotype, their voices are distorted and misunderstood. If she is opinionated, she is difficult. If she speaks with passion, she is volatile. If she explodes with laughter, she is unrefined. If she pitches her neck as she makes a point, she is streetwise and coarse. So much of what Black women say, and how they say it, pushes other people to buy into the myth that Black women are inferior, harsh, and less feminine than other women" (2003, 102). In this same vein, Black women are oppressed at the intersection of their gender and race as they fight against the myth of inferiority and continue to redefine what it means to be Black and a woman in the workplace (Spates et al. 2020). Recently, the COVID-19 pandemic has posed additional workplace challenges and it is important to examine how Black women have been impacted, particularly those in the tech sector. The objective of this study is to understand how Black women make sense of the degree to which the pandemic has been a major catalyst for organizational change, either positively or negatively, which includes how COVID-19 may subsequently impact their workplace experiences and their overall well-being.

Intersectionality Theory and Black Women in the Workplace

To investigate the livelihoods of Black women tech-sector employees before and during COVID-19, I utilized intersectionality theory to conceptualize this study. Kimberlé Crenshaw (1989) created the theoretical framework, intersectionality theory, to depict the ways Black women have been historically marginalized and oppressed within the wider society due to their intersectional identities across gender and race. The compounded effects of racism and sexism adversely impact Black women, wherein they must identify strategies for liberating themselves, one of the central tenets of intersectionality theory (Collins and Bilge 2016; Jordan-Zachery 2007). At the intersection of their gender and race, Black women are subjected to a wide range of discrimination, including critiques or rules about the ways they wear their natural hair in the workplace, being judged by Eurocentric beauty ideals, and workplace bullying, which subsequently affects their career trajectories (Dawson, Karl, and Peluchette 2019; Donahoo and Smith 2019; Hollis 2018). Additionally, Black women are required to code-switch (e.g., change or alter their behaviors) in the workplace because they understand that their intersectional identities are not welcomed by their non-Black colleagues and because their workplace settings are not intended for them to thrive and excel both professionally and personally (Hall et al. 2012; Henry 2000). Thus, some Black women may experience low self-esteem and stress in the workplace due to multiple challenges that they must confront, resist, and overcome (Davis 2019; Hall 2018; Spates et al. 2020).

Overall, the current literature showcases the disparate treatment Black women experience in the workplace due to their identity of being simultaneously Black and woman. Thus, utilizing intersectionality theory to investigate the lived experiences of Black women in the tech sector before and during the COVID-19 pandemic is important for understanding how they have been personally impacted at the intersection of their gender and race and how they navigate and negotiate these challenges. This study is both timely and important given the high stakes for Black women in tech who have been discriminated against, silenced, excluded, and subsequently fired from their tech roles during the COVID-19 pandemic.

Methodology

Qualitative interviews and demographic surveys were collected from Black women currently working in tech organizations across the country. Participants were recruited using social media platforms (e.g., Facebook and Slack groups) and snowball sampling, and recruitment was conducted over a four-week period during the month of November 2020. The research participants' ages range from twenty-four to

TABLE 8.1 Participant Demographic Data

Participant	Age	Employment status	Education status	Geographic region	Current role at tech organization
Olivia	50	Full time	BS	Illinois	Manager
Amelia	32	Full time	MBA	Washington, D.C.	Manager
Mila	24	Full time	BS	Illinois	Analyst
Stella	43	Full time	MA	California	Director
Hazel	24	Full time	BA	California	Diversity strategist
Riley	30	Full time	MBA	California	Marketer

fifty. Table 8.1 provides a detailed overview of the six participants' sociodemographic characteristics. The participants have been in tech from a little less than three years to over twenty years. More information about the research participants is listed in table 8.1 (each participant was given a pseudonym).

Data Collection and Analysis

All of the interviews, conducted via Zoom video conferencing, took roughly fifteen to forty-five minutes to complete. To generate new patterns that materialized during the data analysis process, I used a qualitative research methodology known as grounded theory to interpret the race-gender workplace experiences of Black women in tech careers (Noble and Mitchell 2016; Wiesche et al. 2017). During the data analysis process, I began with extensively familiarizing myself with each interview transcript while listening to the recorded audio portion and creating memos about the participants' similarities and differences as a way to better make sense of the data (Birks, Chapman, and Francis 2008). After examining the interview transcripts, audio recordings, and the notes I drafted during the first round of analysis, I then conducted a second round of analysis of the data and compartmentalized the data to develop and assign new codes (e.g., labels) that emerged from both rounds of data analysis. I then drafted a code-book after the first round of coding to shed light on Black women's workplace experiences in tech, subsequently modifying some codes to adjust for all interview transcript data during the second round of coding. To validate the findings from the study, I utilized several data sources generated from the following activities: (1) conducting a literature review most related to the topic of this current study; (2) writing notes about each participant; (3) conducting an audit train; (4) collecting demographic questionaries; and (5) examining the interview transcript data to both triangulate the data and increase credibility (Leech and Onwuegbuzie 2007; Lincoln and Guba 1986).

Researcher Positionality Statement

I am a Black woman. My research and advocacy work are dedicated to examining and improving the workplace experiences of Black women in science and technology, given the distinct ways in which they are stereotyped and subsequently mistreated. More specifically, I want to ensure that they have safe and inclusive workplace environments that affirm their intersectional identities. As a diversity and inclusion strategist and research scholar, I am well versed on the discriminatory issues (e.g., racism, sexism, elitism, and other isms) that Black women encounter. Black women in America encounter these issues in higher education, their workplaces, and in a variety of other circumstances. In this way, it is important to mention that my intersectional identities across gender and race may have influenced my understanding of the data. As Rogers and Brooms articulate, my "identity locations were relevant for the interview dynamics . . . during data analysis and interpretation" (2019, 449). Overall, this study was conducted to identify the problems Black women tech professionals endure before and during the COVID-19 pandemic, as well as provide some recommendations that tech organizations and companies can utilize to work toward equity and inclusion within the workplace.

Findings and Discussion

Black Women's Workplace Experiences in
Tech Prior to the COVID-19 Pandemic

The first major theme that emerged from the data analysis is that Black women in tech experienced gender and racial discrimination at their places of employment prior to the COVID-19 pandemic. Overall, all of the Black women participants discussed how arduous it is for Black women to enter tech careers. Amelia mentioned that "there are so many requirements . . . that [you have to get before] you can even get an entry-level spot." She added that "they want us to be over-qualified," and "maybe they expect us not to know [as] much or be so easily adaptable." In essence, Amelia articulated two major issues impacting the recruitment process of Black women in the tech sector. One, Black women perceive that they are required to jump through multiple hurdles in order to secure tech positions, unlike their non-Black counterparts. Second, they must combat the functionality of systemic racism and the attendant myth of anti-Black intellectualism ("they expect us to not know as much"). Dating back to chattel slavery, Black people have been typecast as uneducated and their intellect has been repeatedly questioned (Hawkins 2010).

To make matters worse, some of the Black women mentioned that when they, or other Black women, search for employment in the tech sector, they are less likely to receive referrals, and when they do receive referrals, many are still not successful in securing employment. Hazel, who works in a diversity and inclusion strategist role, said, "I referred nearly thirty [Black women] in my four years [at my last job]. And not one of them has ever been hired by the company, not one." Hazel went on to say that "these are [Black] women, who, in many ways, check [all of the] boxes and have the right credentials." These women attended and graduated from "elite universities" and "they still don't get in." The fact that Hazel has recruited close to thirty Black women and not one of them received a job offer is rather troublesome given that the tech sector suffers, historically and contemporarily, from a lack of diversity. Hazel and some other interviewees believe the tech recruiting process involves some level of "unconscious bias," informed by long-standing, systemic racism, that ultimately plagues Black women's chances of entering the tech field.

In addition to identifying multiple and rather abhorrent issues that lessen Black women's chances of pursuing career opportunities in tech, interviewees also expressed that the tech industry can be rather elitist. Amelia said that "a lot of people become elitists." Her reasoning for this evocative statement is that as people in tech continue to move up the career ladder, they forget to help those currently trying to pursue a career in tech. These sentiments were shared by other Black women in this study who expressed that they continuously take it upon themselves to diversify the tech space although it is not in their job descriptions as managers, directors, marketers, and analysts. All six of the participants indicated that they worked to diversify the tech space by providing guidance and mentorship, providing referrals, and by reviewing résumés for Black women and other underrepresented groups.

Given the multiple hurdles Black women must jump through to enter the tech profession, the majority of the women in this study stated they believe that these issues will continue to leave Black women severely underrepresented in tech. This severe underrepresentation causes Black women to experience isolation, a long-standing issue that some of the women in this study have experienced for over twenty years. Olivia mentioned that being the only Black woman (and Black person) in her marketing department constantly leaves her questioning how long will she remain in tech. Olivia recognized that her experience as a Black woman in tech is filled with loneliness, although this is not surprising to her because the tech sector lacks both race and gender diversity in the workplace. As such, her psychological health and well-being is beginning to decline because, as she said, "I think . . . it's starting to weigh on me how lonely the space can be." To be more specific, Olivia has six Black friends who work in the tech sector. However, they all work in "different branches or different professions" and, she expressed, "I never had the experience of having [them] work alongside me." The onliness that Black women are required to experience due to their Blackness and womanhood causes them to question their sense of belonging in predominately white work environments and presents challenges to their overall well-being.

Although all six Black women said they find an overall fulfillment in their job roles, Olivia has also been a recipient of overt racism in the workplace due to the use of the angry Black woman trope by her white woman counterpart, who informed her manger that Olivia was difficult to work with. The manager asked Olivia to "monitor how [she] spoke" to her colleague. This white woman was never asked to change, although her actions were "disruptive" to Olivia and several of her other coworkers. Instead, Olivia had to become "sensitive to her needs" by becoming "more empathetic." Due to the way Olivia was demanded to appease and assuage whiteness in the workplace, she regularly questions whether she was labeled "as the angry Black woman" because, as she stated, "the feedback was a little harsher for me." Not only was Olivia harshly stereotyped as the angry Black woman, but she was also required to code-switch to ensure that her white woman colleague would feel more comfortable around her.

Mila also deals with racism in the workplace, where she is in a leadership role and has a white man reporting directly to her. "He doesn't really listen to me or trust me," she said, "[and] . . . that made me wonder if it's because I'm a Black woman having a white man report to me." The way Mila is adversely impacted by racism leaves her feeling restless and less confident. The biases she spoke to are a reoccurring issue for Black women in the workplace, forcing them to constantly question their ever-present realities (Dickens and Chavez 2018; Walkington 2017). Racism caused some of the Black women who inform this essay to doubt that they experienced some form of prejudice or inequality. Toni Morrison articulates this phenomenon in her speech "A Humanist View," which uniquely positions how racism is a constant and continuous distraction:

> It's important, therefore, to know who the real enemy is, and to know the function, the very serious function of racism, which is distraction. It keeps you from doing your work. It keeps you explaining over and over again, your reason for being. Somebody says you have no language and so you spend 20 years proving that you do. Somebody says your head isn't shaped properly so you have scientists on the fact that it is. Somebody says that you have no art so you dredge that up. Somebody says you have no kingdoms and so you dredge that up. None of that is necessary. (quoted in McKenzie 2014)

The distraction of racism that Toni Morrison speaks to causes marginalized individuals to constantly question and critique themselves. All of the Black women in this study have questioned their positionalities because their mere existence as simultaneously Black and woman presents a problem to some of their colleagues, due to inherent racism and patriarchy at their tech organizations, which is a microcosm of the larger racist society.

Black Women's Workplace Experiences in Tech During COVID-19

The second major theme that emerged is that COVID-19 offered a buffer against the gender and racial discrimination Black women in tech systematically face. All of the Black women interviewed spoke to the benefits of remote working because they no longer had to deal with "casual" forms of race and gender biases that they experienced

prior to COVID-19. Mila, for example, is both hardworking and intelligent but struggles in her leadership position because her colleagues lack respect for her as their superior due to her identity as a
Black woman. Working from home has helped some of these Black
women to "enjoy work more." Olivia's comment best characterizes
how all of the interviewees perceive remote working given the racial
discrimination that has continued to plague the Black community.
She stated, "From a work standpoint . . . I kind of am glad I'm at home
because then I don't have to see people coming up to my face all the
time to see if I'm okay. And I don't know how to really respond. I'm
like, I need you to talk to your uncle, your auntie, your grandma,
and your cousin to tell them to stop killing us. That's what I really
need. Period."

Olivia said she feels that it is vital to her psychological health and
well-being that she continues working remotely. With both COVID-19
and racial injustices running rampant, Olivia's truthful response to her
colleagues' questions about the state of the world is that she wants them
to reflect upon and critique the racism that has been inflicted upon
Black people and other marginalized groups, a process that would begin with their own families. Olivia said she is "thankful" that she can
tell her manager when she is not feeling well due to the continuous
killings of Black women and men, clarifying that she says, "I'm not feeling work today or I'm not here [mentally] but I'm responding intermit-
tently because thinking of being nice right now is just really hard." Not
having to work with their colleagues face-to-face has given all six Black
women the opportunity to focus on their work instead of the overt and
covert racism that is a staple in their workplace environments.[1]

Moreover, by having the opportunity to work remotely, the Black
women described in this essay were able to be their full and complete
selves within the "protected spaces" of their homes. At home, they
can spend their work day in an environment that centers their needs
and where they are treated with respect and dignity. Black women are

able to identify and create comfort within virtual work spaces because their homes have always served as their "comfort zones," safeguarded from the toxicity of their coworkers. These Black women's home spaces are at the intersection of where they need to be and where they want to be. They need and want to be at home because they are never certain about how their non-Black colleagues' behavior will negatively impact them at their places of employment. Thus, the home is where safety and protection are found for Black women in tech.

Despite some relief provided by working at home, Riley has experienced discrimination that adversely impacts her experience working in the tech industry's experiences. Riley said she is "heavily critique[d]": "I have experienced people just dismissing my thoughts [and] my ideas . . . people speak to me in a condescending manner." In addition, she has "experienced gaslighting." These layers of discriminatory treatment leave Riley feeling thrown "off guard" and "stressed out," which causes her to question whether she will remain in tech or pursue another career. Her company shifted to remote working entirely, and Riley understands both the pros and cons of this situation: the pros are that her psychological health and well-being have improved in some areas due to the fact that she no longer has to regularly encounter racism at her physical place of employment, but the cons are that she works much longer hours. At the same time that she experiences some benefit from working remotely, Riley said she experiences declining psychological health and well-being because she is "just expected to do [her] job" despite the constant racial injustices unfolding around her. She explained that she attempts to maintain her sanity by "taking time for [herself] to zone out [and] keeping [herself] busy watching movies." Most importantly, she has been seeking professional therapy, and unplugs from social media by "not logging into Facebook and Instagram" so that she no longer has to watch continuous replays of Black people being murdered. Overall, Black women in tech endure multiple and continuous challenges and stressors as they struggle with barriers to securing employment as well as racism, sexism, and elitism that they experience as full-time employees.

As Black women attempt to find some level of rest in the wake of the COVID-19 pandemic, they are also deeply affected by overlapping racial injustices impacting the Black community. Given that Black people are experiencing a pandemic within a pandemic, some of the Black women interviewed were rather grateful that their tech organizations had personally reached out to them to ask about their experiences, including their psychological health and well-being. Mila mentioned that the director of her company reached out to her multiple times to see how she was faring. Additionally, the company's CEO donated funds "to different Black Lives Matters organizations." "So yeah," she said, "I felt supported from my team members and then also the company as a whole." While Mila felt supported and uplifted as a Black employee at her tech company, other interviewees believed that their organizations were taking part in performative activism—that is, an action "that is done to increase one's social capital rather than because of one's devotion to a cause" (Ashe 2020). Stella said that her experience as a Black woman had not changed during the pandemic even though her tech organization made multiple promises, including, for example, improving hiring practices for Black individuals. Nevertheless, Stella identified "the fact that [her] community is . . . disproportionately impacted by COVID-19" as the single most important issue during these unpredictable and unprecedented times. "That does weigh on me," she said.

The weight that all of the Black women in this study carry is alarming given that they are experiencing declining psychological health and well-being. On top of this burden, Black women are asked to share how their race-gender experiences affect their lived experiences to their non-Black colleagues. Stella articulated the impact that this workplace dynamic has had on her:

In general, I would say, as a Black professional, COVID has not impacted me compared to other groups. However, the fact that these
killings and these murders of Black people has been happening at the
same time—all of a sudden, these companies are aware of how it has
really affected me. Because now people want to talk about it at work,
which is not something I'm used to. I mean, I'm used to talking about
it with other Black people I work with. But I'm not used to being in
a meeting where my white manger is saying, "Black Lives Matters [is
important] and we want to make sure that our Black employees can
bring their full selves to work." That makes me feel a bit uncomfortable.
It makes me question the authenticity of it as well because, why now?
It also adds a weight. Like I almost feel obligated to say something
[and] to speak up. That doesn't feel good. I usually try to take some
distance from it.

Stella's reflection signifies how emotionally heavy COVID-19 and overlapping police brutality has been for the Black women interviewed.
She said that she is not personally impacted by COVID-19 but she indeed is personally impacted because her workplace has made her uncomfortable. She is left attempting to figure out why major tech companies are now worried about how Black people have historically been
treated. Having these race-related conversations about anti-Blackness
while at work is emotionally exhausting for Stella because it "adds a
weight"—she feels that she has to speak up about the racial and social
injustices that are negatively impacting the Black community, but she
understands the relative importance of distancing herself from the
"weight" and heaviness of these conversations, especially in the workplace. Similarly, Olivia regularly questions the tech industry's ulterior
motives: "I haven't seen any change from any of these tech companies
that actually have the power to do it. . . . a lot of the organizations
that I've been working with have made concerted efforts to be more
vocal about what's going on. I will say that I hesitate and that I am not

sure that I trust their messages, which makes me feel guarded." She expressed that change can be made but that certain tech companies are unwilling to enact change that is crucial for the recruitment and retention of Black people in the tech sector. Although many tech firms are committing to diversifying their organizations, Olivia mentioned that they were "under-hiring [before COVID] anyway, so you're not necessarily doing anything equitable from the jump," leading her to believe that they will continue to under-hire racially underrepresented groups although they have published public statements suggesting otherwise. The power and privilege endemic in under-hiring speaks directly to how white supremacy is upheld.

Olivia's thoughts are similar to those of Riley, who says that the tech industry does not care about their Black employees. For example, Riley mentioned that her company created the Black Employee Resource Group (ERG) to support Black employees only. She shared, "[They ask us to] say a few words so that we can say 'Black Lives Matter.' And I've been pulled into that and then there are times where I've had people who were scared to talk because they know what's happening in society, but they don't know how to approach me." Riley is also confused by the fact that her non-Black colleagues are "hesitant" to have conversations about anti-Blackness. Riley thinks "it's concerning how some folks [are just] oblivious [about issues of racism] or they don't want to talk it." The outright privilege of Riley's non-Black colleagues who are complicit and comfortable in being "oblivious" about racism within the wider society, and who have no desire to learn about it, leave Black women such as Riley feeling vulnerable, depressed, and defenseless. Unfortunately, all of the Black women who were interviewed felt that they have little choice but to speak about issues of racial prejudice that affect their lived experiences—and the experiences of the larger Black community—as the nation attempts to reckon with these public health and social problems. Riley concluded that "it's shooting season for people like me and we are in lots of trouble. [There are people] who are bold about their racism and their prejudice and it's just so scary to see how it is played out on TV and in the media." This leaves her unsure of whether she should be vocal about Black Lives Matter at her place of employment or keep things business as usual: She does not want to be the spokesperson for the entire race and she experiences, as do many people, racial battle fatigue from seeing Black people killed on television and various social media platforms. This repetitious murder imagery traumatizes them and reminds them of the hurt, harm, and danger that affects the livelihoods of Black people historically and contemporarily.

Racial discrimination is "both a mental and public health crisis" (Spencer 2021, 1) that impacts Black people (Garcia and Sharif 2015; Laurencin and Walker 2020). Psychologically and physiologically burdened by the various ways they are discriminated against, the Black women who inform this study do not want to be the spokesperson on behalf of their race in the workplace. They do not want to share their pain to ensure that their non-Black colleagues more closely understand the consequences of racism and sexism. They do not want to take on diversity and inclusion roles just because they are Black women. Instead, they desire for their tech organizations to create equitable recruitment and retention practices that will ensure that Black people and other underrepresented groups are better represented in the tech field as they have promised during this pandemic. They desire to be respected in the workplace. Tech organizations must protect Black employees as they grapple with the effects of COVID-19 and overlapping racial injustices.

Conclusion: Black Women in the Tech Sector Before and During COVID-19

The racism and sexism that Black women in the tech sector encounter is both deplorable and deeply engrained. Black women experience prejudice and must contend with various stereotypes, such as the angry Black woman, and the myth of Black anti-intellectualism. Additionally, they are ignored and silenced in the workplace and must code-switch in order to appease and assuage whiteness even if they hold leadership positions. The disparate treatment that they experience in tech causes them to repeatedly question why various tech organizations and companies are now wanting to address racism and recruit and retain more Black employees. Given the broader impacts of both COVID-19 and racial injustices on Black individuals, it becomes an additional burden on Black women when they are tapped to share their lived experiences in the United States. Black women are left stuck in a difficult position because they desire to liberate Black people but are psychologically exhausted by these types of conversations and do not want to share the associative trauma that they carry. Black women question the motives of their companies and feel upset and hurt that their organizations appear to be participating in performative activism rather than enacting substantive change.

The power and privilege that is deeply associated with and entrenched within the role of performative activism in tech, which ranges from press releases to hiring goals to diversity and inclusion efforts, silences and excludes underrepresented groups that have been historically marginalized. Performative activism without corrective action leaves employees, such as the Black women discussed here, mentally exhausted and disappointed. In order to create systemic change, we must first understand that activism is not a trend and that to engage meaningfully, we must hold organizations and companies accountable to ensure that they actually take steps toward the changes they described.

For example, an important finding from this study is that remote working was found to better support Black women because it affords them self-protected spaces (e.g., their homes) that can shield them from the racism and sexism they would normally experience in the physical workplace. In addition, they are more comfortable in a virtual space because it gives them greater ability to exercise agency and control over the types of race-related conversations they will have or not have with their colleagues. This enables Black women to actually focus on their work instead of gender and racial discrimination or being asked to be the spokesperson of the Black experience as it relates to the ongoing killings of Black people at the hands of police officers. Remote working may be the future trend since some companies are beginning to realize that workers can be more productive at home and there are fewer overhead costs. Beyond this immediately obvious material benefit, it is important that companies also understand that working from home may be psychologically safer for groups that have been marginalized. Companies now have the opportunity to begin or continue to create an ecosystem (e.g., inclusive and diverse environment) that is not deeply embedded within systemic racism, sexism, and elitism as their employees work from home. To this end, I offer several recommendations that tech companies can use to support and uplift Black women employees:

1. Supervisors should regularly ask Black women how the company can best support them in the workplace to help ensure their success and longevity in the field.

2. In all efforts to create and sustain a safe and inclusive workplace environment, management should center and validate Black women's workplace experiences across their various intersectional identities.

3. All employees should be required to enroll in and complete diversity-related training and supervisors should follow up with their staff and ask them what they learned through their participation, including how they can apply what they learned to effect positive change within the workplace.

4. Tech organizations must understand that it is not solely up to Black women to diversify the tech field. Diversity strategists should be hired that promote inclusive recruitment and hiring practices to attract more Black professionals to tech.

5. Tech organizations need to disengage from performative activism and instead focus on creating sustainable changes that benefit Black professionals.

Altogether, tech companies have a great deal of work ahead of them as they endeavor to create safe spaces for their Black employees and diversify the field.

Note

1. Interestingly, other studies have found that Black remote workers in the tech sector claim that they are experiencing more discrimination across race and gender lines than when they worked in person at their places of employment (Project Include 2021).

Bibliography

Alegria, Sharla N. 2020. "What Do We Mean by Broadening Participation? Race, Inequality, and Diversity in Tech Work." *Sociology Compass* 14, no. 6 (March): 1–12. https://doi.org/10.1111/soc4.12793.

Ashe, Lauren. 2020. "The Dangers of Performative Activism." VOX ATL, June 23, 2020. https://voxatl.org/the-dangers-of-performative-activism/.

Atewologun, Doyin, Ruth Sealy, and Susan Vinnicombe. 2015. "Revealing Intersectional Dynamics in Organizations Introducing 'Intersectional Identity Work.'" *Gender, Work and Organization* 23, no. 3 (April): 223–47. https://doi.org/10.1111/gwao.12082.

Birks, Melanie, Ysanne Chapman, and Karen Francis. 2008. "Memoing in Qualitative Research: Probing Data and Processes." *Journal of Nursing in Research* 13, no. 1 (January): 68–75. https://doi.org/10.1177/1744987107081254.

Collins, Patricia Hill, and Sirma Bilge. 2016. *Intersectionality*. Cambridge, U.K.: Polity Press.

Condon, Stephanie. 2020. "Approximately 117,000 IT Jobs Lost Since March, US Data Shows." ZDNet, June 5, 2020. https://www.zdnet.com/article/it-jobs-lost/.

Crenshaw, Kimberlé. 1989. "Demarginalizing the Intersection of Race and Sex: A Black Feminist Critique of Antidiscrimination Doctrine, Feminist Theory and Antiracist Politics." *University of Chicago Legal Forum* 1989, no. 1: 139–67. https://chicagounbound.uchicago.edu/uclf/vol1989/iss1/8.

Davis, Gena Y. 2019. "The Self-Esteem of Black Female Corporate Professionals in the Workplace: How Unconscious and Implicit Bias Played a Role." PhD diss., Alliant International University. https://www.proquest.com/openview /4b8df84e4cceb630da68233829cea27f/1?pq-origsite=gscholarandcbl=18750 anddiss=y.

Dawson, Gail A., Katherine A. Karl, and Joy V. Peluchette. "Hair Matters: Toward Understanding Natural Hair Bias in the Workplace." 2019. *Journal of Leadership and Organizational Studies* 26, no. 3 (August): 389–401. https:// doi.org/10.1177/1548051819848998.

Dickens, Danielle, Maria Jones, and Naomi Hall. 2020. "Being a Token Black Female Faculty Member in Physics: Exploring Research on Gendered Racism, Identity Shifting as a Coping Strategy, and Inclusivity in Physics." *Physics Teacher* 50: 335–37. https://doi.org/10.1119/1.5145529.

Dickens, Danielle D., and Ernest L. Chavez. 2018. "Navigating the Workplace: The Costs and Benefits of Shifting Identities at Work Among Early Career U.S. Black Women." *Sex Roles* 78: 760–74. https://doi.org/10.1007/s11199-017 -0844-x.

Dickens, Danielle D., Veronica Y. Womack, and Treshae Dimes. 2019. "Managing Hypervisibility: An Exploration of Theory and Research on Identity Shifting Strategies in the Workplace Among Black Women." *Journal of Vocational Behavior* 113 (August): 153–63. https://doi.org/10.1016/j.jvb.2018.10.008.

Donahoo, Saran, and Asia D. Smith. 2019. "Controlling the Crown: Legal Efforts to Professionalize Black Hair." *Race and Justice* 12, no. 1 (November): 182–203. https://doi.org/10.1177/2153368719888264.

Donovan, Roxanne A., David J. Glaban, Ryan K. Grace, Jacqueline K. Bennet, and Shaina Z. Felicie. 2012. "Impact of Racial Macro- and Microaggressions in Black Women's Lives: A Preliminary Analysis." *Journal of Black Psychology* 39, no. 2: 185–96. https://doi.org/10.1177/0095798412443259.

Erete, Sheena, Yolanda A. Rankin, and Jakita O. Thomas. 2020. "I Can't Breathe: Reflections from Black Women in CSCW and HCI." *Proceedings of the ACM on Human-Computer Interaction* 4, no. 3: 1–23. https://doi.org/10.1145/3432933.

Gamst, Glenn, Leticia Arellano-Morales, Lawrence S. Meyers, Dylan G. Serpas, Jessica Balla, Angelica Diaz, Kaycee Dobson, et al. 2020. "Shifting Can Be Stressful for African American Women: A Structural Mediation Model."

Journal of Black Psychology 46, no. 5 (July): 364–87. https://doi.org/10.1177 /0095798420939721.

Garcia, Jennifer L., and Mienah Z. Sharif. 2015. "Black Lives Matter: A Commentary on Racism and Public Health." *American Journal of Public Health* 105, no. 8 (August): 27–30. https://doi.org/10.2105/AJPH.2015.302706.

Hague, LaShanda Y., and Comfort O. Okpala. 2017. "Voices of African American Women Leaders on Factors That Impact Their Career Advancement in North Carolina Community Colleges." *Journal of Research Initiatives* 2, no. 3: 1–9. https://digitalcommons.uncfsu.edu/jri/vol2/iss3/3.

Hall, Camille J. 2018. "It Is Tough Being a Black Woman: Intergenerational Stress and Coping." *Journal of Black Studies* 49, no. 5 (July): 481–501. https:// doi.org/10.1177/0021934718766817.

Hall, Camille J., Joyce C. Everett, and Johnnie Hamilton-Mason. 2012. "Black Women Talk About Workplace Stress and How They Cope." *Journal of Black Studies* 43, no. 2 (March): 207–26. https://doi.org/10.1177%2F0021934711413272.

Hawkins, Billy. 2010. *The New Plantation: Black Athletes, College Sports, and Predominately White NCAA Institutions.* New York: Palgrave Macmillan.

Henry, Annette. 2000. "Thoughts on Black Women in the Workplace: A Space Not Intended for Us." *Urban Education* 35, no. 5 (December), 520–24. https:// doi.org/10.1177/0042085900355002.

Hollis, Leah P. 2018. "Bullied Out of the Position: Black Women's Complex Intersectionality, Workplace Bullying, and Resulting Career Disruption." *Journal of Black Sexuality and Relationships* 4, no. 3 (Winter): 73–89. https:// doi.org/10.1353/bsr.2018.0004.

Huisache, Sam. 2020. "The Impact of COVID-19 on Women in Tech." Trust-Radius, May 11, 2020. https://www.trustradius.com/vendor-blog/covid-19 -women-in-tech.

Iheduru-Anderson, Kechi. 2020. "Barriers to Career Advancement in the Nursing Profession: Perceptions of Black Nurses in the United States." *Nursing Forum* 55, no. 4 (July): 664–77. https://doi.org/10.1111/nuf.12483.

Jones, Charisse, and Shorter-Gooden, Kumea. 2003. *Shifting: The Double Lives of Black Women in America.* New York: HarperCollins.

Jordan-Zachery, Julia S. 2007. "Am I a Black Woman or a Woman Who Is Black? A Few Thoughts on the Meaning of Intersectionality." *Critical Perspectives* 3, no. 2 (June): 254–63. https://doi.org/10.1017/S1743923X07000074.

Laurencin, Cato L., and Joanne M. Walker. 2020. "A Pandemic on a Pandemic: Racism and COVID-19 in Blacks." *Cell Systems* 11, no. 1 (July): 9–10. https:// doi.org/10.1016%2Fj.cels.2020.07.002.

Leech, Nancy L., and Anthony J. Onwuegbuzie. 2007. "An Array of Qualitative Data Analysis Tools: A Call for Data Analysis Triangulation." *School Psychology Quarterly* 22, no. 4 (December): 557–83. http://dx.doi.org/10.1037 /1045-3830.22.4.557.

Lincoln, Yvonna S., and Egon G. Guba. 1986. "But Is It Rigorous? Trustworthiness and Authenticity in Naturalistic Evaluation." *New Directions for Program Evaluation* 1986, no. 30 (Summer): 73–84. https://doi.org/10.1002/ev.1427.

McKenzie, Keisha. 2014. "Transcript: Toni Morrison at Portland State University, 1975." *MacKenzian* (blog), July 7, 2014. https://mackenzian.com/blog /2014/07/07/transcript-morrison-1975/.

Noble, Helen, and Gary Mitchell. 2016. "What Is Grounded Theory?" *Evidence-Based Nursing* 19: 34–35. http://dx.doi.org/10.1136/eb-2016-102306.

Project Include. 2021. "Remote Work Since Covid-19 Is Exacerbating Harm: What Companies Need to Know and Do." https://projectinclude.org/remote -work-report/.

Rankin, Yolanda A., and Jakita O. Thomas. 2020. "The Intersectional Experiences of Black Women in Computing." *Proceedings of the 51st ACM Technical Symposium on Computer Science Education (SIGSCE)*: 199–205. https://doi .org/10.1145/3328778.3366873.

Reynolds-Dobbs, Wendy, Kecia M. Thomas, and Matthew S. Harrison. 2008. "From Mammy to Superwoman: Images That Hinder Black Women's Career Development." *Journal of Career Development* 35, no. 2: 129–50. https://doi .org/10.1177/0894845308325645.

Rogers, Leoandra Onnie, and Derrick R. Brooms. 2019. "Ideology and Identity Among White Male Teachers in an All-Black, All-Male High School." *American Educational Research Journal* 57, no. 1 (June): 440–70. https://doi.org /10.3102%2F0002831219853224.

Spates, Kamesha, Na'Tasha M. Evans, Brittany C. Watts, Nasra Abubakar, and Tierra James. 2020. "Keeping Ourselves Sane: A Qualitative Exploration of Black Women's Coping Strategies for Gendered Racism." *Sex Roles* 82: 513–24. https://doi.org/10.1007/s11199-019-01077-1.

Spencer, Breauna Marie. 2021. "The Psychological Costs of Experiencing Racial Discrimination in the Ivory Tower: The Untold Stories of Black Men Enrolled in Science, Technology, Engineering, and Mathematics (STEM) Doctoral Programs." *Sociological Forum* 36, no. 3 (September): 1–23. https:// doi.org/10.1111/socf.12724.

Thomas, Jakita, Nicole Joseph, Arian Williams, Chant'el Crum, and Jamika Burge. 2018. "Speaking Truth to Power: Exploring the Intersectional Experiences of Black Women in Computing." *2018 Research on Equity and Sus-*

tained Participation in Engineering, Computing, and Technology (RESPECT): 1–8. https://doi.org/10.1109/RESPECT.2018.8491718.

Walkington, Lori. 2017. "How Far Have We Really Come? Black Women Faculty and Graduate Students' Experiences in Higher Education." *Humboldt Journal of Social Relation* 1, no. 39: 51–65. https://doi.org/10.55671/0160-4341.1022.

Wiesche, Manuel, Marlen C. Jurisch, Phillip W. Yetton, and Helmut Krcmar. 2017. "Grounded Theory Methodology in Information Systems Research." *MIS Quarterly* 41, no. 3: 685–701. https://doi.org/10.25300/MISQ%2F2017%2F41.3.02.

Wingfield, Adia Harvey, and Renée Skeete Alston. 2014. "Maintaining Hierarchies in Predominately White Organizations: A Theory of Racial Tasks." *American Behavioral Scientist* 58, no. 2 (July): 274–87. https://doi.org/10.1177%2F0002764213503329.

Fugitive Breath, Breathing Bones

Ancestral Guide for Abolishing Anti-Black Gendered COVID-19 Necropolitics

Shamara Wyllie Alhassan

We all begin life in water
We all begin life because someone once breathed for us
Until we breathe for ourselves
Someone breathes for us
Everyone has had someone—a woman—breathe for them
Until that first ga(s)p
For air

—M. NourbeSe Philip, "The Ga(s)p"

Our deaths inside a system of racism existed before we were born.

—Claudia Rankine, "The Condition of Black Life Is One of Mourning"

Fugitive Breathing Through Anti-Black Gendered COVID-19 Necropolitics

Air . . . Breathe . . .
Inhale . . . Exhale . . .
Inhale . . . Exhale . . .
Inhale . . . Exhale . . .
Feel the air move in through your nostrils and out through your
slightly open lips.

Deeply expand and contract your lungs. Feel the rise and fall of your
   gentle life's breath.
Cherish this breathing.
In this moment.
At this time.

How Do Bones Breathe?

Breathing, which is the very core of living, changed after the onset of
COVID-19. We were required to wear masks, and when we contracted
COVID, we had to lie on our stomachs to breathe (Thompson et al.
2020). Some of us did not survive this new way of breathing and transitioned to the ancestral realm; some lived and harmed themselves or
others; and some found ways to cope with illness, adapt to physical
distance, and breathe through social justice advocacy. How can a reflection on the ways breathing transformed during COVID provide
an opportunity to envision anew breathing in a COVID world? How
do we reflect on being socially close, even while maintaining physical
distance? M. NourbeSe Philip writes about breath as a radical hospitality that grounds us in "a model of community and connectedness in
a more female-centered, embodied symbolic universe" (2018, 36). She
theorizes her notion of breath through the physiological development
of a fetus in a mother's womb. To be in the womb of someone who
carries us is to be completely dependent upon someone else. This sacred circular breath imprinted on the memory of every human is the
beginning of interconnectedness or sociogeny, as Frantz Fanon (2008)
would put it. Sociogeny recognizes that human beings are relational.
We are meant to be in relation to other humans, not only to each other
but to the ancestors and the environment, and we become who we are
in this relation, as part of the circular and reciprocal relationship that
we were nurtured by in the wombs of our mothers. But something
happens as we grow and structures of oppression disconnect us from

our relational beingness. We become individuals gasping for breath, like the first gasp we take on our own after being birthed into the world or our last gasp before death. Flowing from our mothers, we explode into our own personhood, but we still maintain that dependency, that need for relation. At what point do we forget this need for circular breath or relation?

Fugitive breath[1] recognizes that we live in a world where breathing while Black is criminalized; therefore, the very act of breathing while Black is a subversive and fugitive act and can become a guide to survival and freedom. Fugitive breathing as a guide for survival focuses our attention to the sequelae that reverberates from the families, friends, and communities of those who have transitioned to the ancestral realm. Fugitive breath recognizes the continuity and fluidity of life in multiple formations. Working in the Africana spiritual traditions of Rastafari and La Regla de Ocha, fugitive breath insists on life in its multiplicity and enacts a mourning of the physical temple that housed the spirit of those we have lost but celebrates the enduring ancestral future that our dead prepare for us. Living and breathing with our ancestors undoes the necropolitics of the state by rejecting its power to let live or let die.

Drawing from Achille Mbembe's (2003) notion of necropolitics, which is the power of the state to let live, let die, or keep the body in pain, Christen Smith's (2016) concept of anti-Black gendered necropolitics names the reverberating undocumented health effects that Black families continue to live with during and after the initial murder of a Black person. I contend that COVID-19 exacerbated the anti-Black gendered necropolitics that Smith theorizes. Therefore, I offer the term *anti-Black gendered COVID-19 necropolitics*, which links the pandemic of COVID-19 to the pandemic of white supremacy, anti-Black genocide, and the continued reverberating racial trauma experienced by Black families. Recently, there have been studies that use the lens of necropolitics to understand the multiple pandemics of COVID-19, white supremacy, racial capitalism, and state murder, but studies have not yet considered the disproportionate epidemiological impacts of COVID-19 and anti-Black gendered necropolitics (Sandset 2021).

Sitting with death and still breathing becomes a fugitive act, a radical praxis that rewrites the campaigns of necropower by insisting upon our living. There is a long-standing anti-Black belief that Black lungs are faulty and cannot draw oxygen in the ways that other racialized lungs can (Braun 2014). Black women breathing with the full expansion of their lungs abolishes anti-Black physiology, and during COVID-19, their breathing questions the way we treat an airborne illness that impacts the lungs. Black women breathing, witnessing, writing, and speaking themselves into narratives that would abort their being contradicts anti-Black mythological narratives that suggest Black people are genetically predisposed to being infected by COVID-19, by exposing the very institutions responsible for care as the progenitors of death (Gravlee 2020).

I offer the narrative of Dr. Susan Moore as an important example of the ways Black women advocated for themselves in the midst of COVID-19 and racist medical treatment. Born in Jamaica and raised in Michigan, Dr. Moore was a Black physician who chronicled her battle with racism on a Facebook video after her COVID-19 diagnosis (Democracy Now! 2020). In her social media post, Moore discussed the ways her pain was disregarded by doctors because they made her feel like a drug addict for requesting pain medication. At each stage of her hospital stay, from breathing trouble to physical pain to the denial of basic treatments for COVID-19, Moore had to advocate for herself. When the hospital decided to discharge her prematurely, she noted that was the way medical facilities murdered Black people. "This is how Black people get killed, when you send them home and they don't know how to fight for themselves . . . I had to talk to somebody, maybe the media, somebody, to let people know how I'm being treated in this place" (Mack 2020). Moore died on December 20, 2020, three weeks after her COVID-19 diagnosis. She is survived by her son, Henry Muhammed, who was nineteen years old at the time of her death (Adams 2021).

The *New York Times* reported that Moore's death and her choice to share her experiences have elevated the issue of racial disparities in the ways Black patients are treated compared to their white counterparts (Eligon 2020). After Moore died, Indiana University Health North (IU Health North), the hospital delivering adverse care to Moore, investigated her allegations. IU Health North president and CEO Dennis Murphy issued a statement that found while there was no technical malpractice in terms of her medical care, the medical staff did not take the time to hear and understand her concerns (Rudavsky 2021). An external investigation into Dr. Moore's claims of racist health-care treatment found that she received proper care but acknowledged the health-care providers' lack of cultural competency in delivering care (Rudavsky 2021). While institutional investigations are important, their credibility in this case is called into question by what Dr. Moore said she experienced before she died. Attending to the qualitative experiences of Black women receiving racist medical care and foregrounding restorative justice is an appropriate response to claims of harm. While denials may save institutions from lawsuits, they do not provide moral accountability or uphold the Hippocratic oath medical professionals take.

Throughout the pandemic, the under-resourced nature of health-care infrastructure globally led to a massive shortage of personal protective equipment (PPE) (Burki 2020, 785–86). Health-care professionals could not adequately protect themselves against the airborne virus. The lack of PPE for medical professionals combined with limited knowledge of what the novel coronavirus was, how it spread, and how to treat it, plus preexisting racial inequities in medical care, spelled death for Black and Brown people. Ostensibly, these extenuating circumstances may be considered when assessing IU Health North's culpability, but the admission that health-care providers lacked cultural competence begs the question of how medical professionals can adequately treat illness without having a foundation in racial health disparities and the ability to hear, understand, and respond to patient concerns and questions (Health Justice Commons n.d.).

IU Health North is not singular in its disregard of Black women's questions and concerns. Medical professionals are usually responsive to apparent physical ailments, but holistic care involves attending to the physical, emotional, psychological, and spiritual lives of patients. Holistic care is critical during COVID-19 because the epidemiology of the virus is still unfolding and medical professionals are learning best practices for treating, preventing, and mitigating the effect of the virus. Holistic care takes time, is anti-capitalist, is humane, and demands anti-racist competency, compassion, and a fundamental consideration of the way structural issues impact health. Holistic care is an important first step to responding to enduring anti-Black gendered COVID-19 necropolitics and must be addressed as the global pandemic rages and the vaccine apartheid between over-resourced countries and under-resourced countries widens (Lanziotti et al. 2022). Until we have holistic care, we rely on our fugitive breath and insist on life even in the face of medical industries designed to foment our demise.

The American Medical Association (AMA) released its most comprehensive diagnostic report of the long-standing problem of white supremacy and the systemic effects of racism in the medical field, both in terms of racial disparities in care for patients and in discrimination against Black doctors and other medical professionals (AMA 2021). As a Black woman and a physician, Dr. Moore stood at the apex of these overlapping concerns. While the AMA's detailed plan to address racial inequities is important, it is too late for Dr. Moore. Invoking anti-Black gendered COVID-19 necropolitics allows us to not lose sight of the premeditated nature of public health facilities when it comes to enacting necropolitical logics.

Racial trauma should be considered a component of COVID symptoms that medical professionals treat. The Centers for Disease Control and Prevention (CDC) in the United States reported that Black and Brown people have increased risk of getting COVID-19 and experiencing severe illness or death. Reasons for increased risk include racial disparities in health care, frontline-worker status with high social contact, and comorbidities or underlying health conditions (CDC 2020a). Black women have increased vulnerabilities due to complications with long-term COVID symptoms and racism among medical professionals, which can lead to premature death (Fadulu 2022; Cooney 2021; Rushovich and Richardson 2021). COVID-19 exposed and exacerbated the lack of commitment to holistic health-care solutions for ailing patients and amplified the long history of Black women's concerns being disregarded by medical professionals. While the epidemiology of coronavirus continues to unfold, noting gendered and racial inequities in contracting, being severely impacted by, and dying of COVID-19 is critical to understanding the virus.

There are enduring physical symptoms of COVID-19 like difficulty breathing or shortness of breath, fatigue, chronic pain, depression or anxiety, and other neurological issues that linger far beyond the initial diagnosis of COVID (Mayo Clinic Staff 2022). Some COVID-19 patients that experience these symptoms for more than six months "meet the diagnostic criteria" for myalgic encephalomyelitis/chronic fatigue syndrome (ME/CFS), which is a long-term illness that "sometimes follows a viral illness and leads to long-term pain, fatigue, and other symptoms that can last decades" and that "primarily affected upper-class white women" (Ducharme 2021). Black women have mobilized for decades to change the association of ME/CFS with white women. Advocates like Wilhelmina Jenkins fought to receive a diagnosis for their ME/CFS and helped get the CDC to recognize that people of color also suffer with this illness (Ducharme 2021). However, people of color are still not represented adequately in research on the condition (Ducharme 2021). Some patients experiencing long COVID may not have been tested for COVID-19 due to inadequate testing resources at the beginning of the pandemic, but their enduring symptoms can lead to a diagnosis of long COVID. About 10 percent to 30 percent of COVID-19 patients are designated as long-haulers (Rubin 2020).

In 2021, then director of the National Institutes of Health (NIH) in the United States, Francis S. Collins, announced a $1.15 billion NIH initiative, funded by the U.S. Congress, for four years of research into the causes, long-term effects, potential treatments, and preventions of long COVID, officially referred to as Post-Acute Sequelae of SARS-CoV-2 infection (PASC) (Collins 2021). While data concerning long COVID is still evolving, research indicates that long-term illness may be more prevalent in women (Sudre et al. 2021). Taking these preliminary research results together with the fact that COVID-19 adversely impacts Black people, there is a high probability that a sizeable percentage of Black women are experiencing long-term COVID-19 symptoms.

Describing herself on her website as "an intuitive, mouthy, and disagreeable woman who breathed the wrong air one day" (Smith n.d.) thirty-eight-year-old Chimére L. Smith, a patient advocate and consultant for Black long-COVID patients in urban communities, recounts being accused of being a drug user or dismissed as mentally ill when seeking help from medical professionals due to her long-COVID symptoms. "I've had some doctors accuse me of being aggressive. I've been asked about drug use more times than I ever care to recall. As a woman and as a Black woman, I understand the history of discrimination when it comes to healthcare in this country, but I never really quite knew until it knocked on my door" (Ducharme 2021). Rather than remain silent about her experiences or accept racist medical assumptions, Smith became one of the first Black woman to testify before "the House Committee on Energy and Commerce's hearing on long COVID" about Black women and long COVID-19 (Smith 2021). In her April 2021 testimony, she said,

> There is growing evidence of the direct connection between myalgic encephalomyelitis and Long COVID, we must reconcile that our unwillingness to recognize chronic conditions we can't visibly see has contributed to generations of black people who have already disappeared from society . . . I speak now so I am not just another disabled black woman in America carrying the sorrow, humiliation, and pain of this and other conditions on my shoulders. I speak now so my former students can access comprehensive education and treatment for Long COVID years after this is no longer a trending topic. (Smith 2021)

Smith's witnessing of her own experiences helps to place Black women as central to developing the epidemiologic profile of long COVID and exposes the long-term generational traumas of being Black, woman, and disabled in the United States. Smith's testimony ensures that other Black people with chronic disabilities will not have to fight so hard to be heard and treated equitably when they seek medical assistance. In a video segment produced by the *Washington Post*, Jameta Nicole Barlow, a community health psychologist, commented, "If you are a healthcare professional, you need to treat every Black girl or woman who walks into your room as if they're someone whose experience is worthy of you listening to, recognizing their full humanity, because too often they've sat in those exam rooms and they haven't been heard" (Sitz 2021). While a clear definition of long COVID is still materializing, what is clear is that racial inequity is a major indicator of who is able to be diagnosed and treated for long COVID. Dr. Moore's premature death and Smith's discriminatory treatment illustrate the ways Black women are at a severe disadvantage when seeking care for COVID. I lift up their stories as central to understanding the racial trauma and epidemiology of COVID-19 on Black women and their families. Attention to anti-Black gendered COVID-19 necropolitics provides a framework for health-care providers to understand their role in deciding who recovers, who lives in enduring pain without treatment, and who dies because of the interwoven anti-Blackness that pervades all aspects of the health-care system. Black women's personal narratives articulate a vision where the guarantee of death transforms into one of life through breathing, being breathed for, and breathing for our ancestors.

Breathing Bones as Ancestral Guide for Freedom

Breathing provides a fugitive guide to surviving the constant push toward death, the Black corpses inured to our living, the lingering grief, trauma, and illness that characterizes constant loss of loved ones and the consistent terror that sutures Black existence. Meditating on the notion of cyclical breath, I realized we breathe in fugitivity through our insistence on witnessing, mourning, and envisioning new futures. Occurring in both the material and the metaphysical realms, this fugitive breath challenges state logics of death. Anti-Black gendered COVID-19 necropolitics reveals the ways the dead haunt us. Our past is made present through the constant witnessing, documenting, and fugitive breathing of our ancestral bones. Many have described 2020 as a year of racial reckoning. But a reckoning requires acknowledgement, atonement, reparations, and justice.

The year 2020 has been a year of our dead breathing themselves into the present. Hearing the spring 2021 developments regarding the MOVE bombing victims of 1985 showed me that the dead themselves, as copresent beings from the spiritual realm, can breathe with us and offer their own legacy to expose the depths of anti-Black genocide and white supremacy (Kassutto 2021). On May 13, 1985, the home of MOVE, a Black liberation organization, was bombed by the Philadelphia Police Department in broad daylight after a decade of antagonism between the organization and the City, stoked in large part by former mayor Frank L. Rizzo's targeted campaign to eradicate MOVE during the 1970s (Roane 2021). The city's fire department, for over an hour, did nothing to stop the ensuing fire from the bomb and police shot at MOVE members who tried to escape the fire, resulting in a horrific scene: "Although Ramona [Africa] and one child, Birdie Africa, survived the catastrophic fire, in total 11 MOVE members including five children, as well as their dogs, perished. More than 250 others in the Cobbs Creek neighborhood were displaced when the fire destroyed 50 neighboring rowhomes" (Roane 2021). The bombing of MOVE was catastrophic for the Black community in Philadelphia and exercised the anti-Black genocidal politics of the U.S. government just sixty-four years after the 1921 Tulsa massacre (Roberts 2021). On November 12, 2020, the Philadelphia City Council finally apologized for the 1985 MOVE bombing (McCrystal 2020).

In April 2021, a story broke that the bones of the victims bombed at the MOVE headquarters were being housed at the University of Pennsylvania (Penn) and later were transferred and used in an online course on physical anthropology at Princeton University (Kassutto 2021). Apparently, the remains had been in the custody of Alan Mann, a university professor who is now retired—they were given to him to identify and when he was not able to conclusively identify them, they were not repatriated to the MOVE family, even though they had been positively identified as the MOVE children by another physical anthropologist (Flaherty 2021a). The bones belong to two little girls, Katricia "Tree" Africa and Zanetta Dotson Africa, who were fourteen and twelve when they were murdered by the City of Philadelphia (Kassutto 2021). Penn and Princeton have issued apologies and said they are working on repatriating the remains (Flaherty 2021b). The indiscriminate use of the bones to educate future physical anthropologists illustrates the ways our educational institutions and our government completely disregard the long-term traumas of Black families, disrespect the remains of the racialized dead, and use the bodies of murdered children to teach anti-Blackness to the next generation.

The MOVE family continues to demand justice. Mike Africa Jr., a current member of the MOVE organization, was shocked and disturbed by the news that his relatives had been denied a resting place. "They were bombed, and burned alive," Africa Jr. said, "and now you wanna keep their bones" (Kassutto 2021). Consuewella Dotson Africa, the mother of Tree Africa, recently passed away at the Hospital of the University of Pennsylvania due, in part, to stress after the news of the location and use of her daughter's remains surfaced in April 2021 (Goodin-Smith and Dean 2021). Speaking of Consuewella Africa's death, Janine Africa, another MOVE member, told the *Philadelphia Inquirer*, "She was exposed to COVID, but she had gotten over COVID, and the doctors were saying she started having lung problems, and they were saying it was because of stress. That's understandable" (Goodin-Smith and Dean 2021). During a news conference in April concerning the mishandling of her daughter's remains, Consuewella Africa told reporters, "I mean, it's just continuous, nonstop, vicious, violent, sadistic, ongoing abuse of the MOVE organization.... Why? Because we stand up and tell the truth about this rotten reformed world system" (Goodin-Smith and Dean 2021). There are no words to express the horror of knowing that the bones of your children are, as Mike Africa Jr. put it, "being played with" (Goodin-Smith and Dean 2021) by so-called scholars for decades after the state murdered them. These bones evidence the continued breathing of our ancestors, placing this case back in our collective moral consciousness.

When Achille Mbembe (2003) theorized necropolitics, he spoke about the power of the state to let live or let die, but also the power of the state to keep people's bodies in pain. This chronic pain combined with the global pandemic of COVID-19 clearly compromised Consuewella Africa's health in a hyper-weathering effect. Arline Geronimus et al. (2006) have shown that repeated encounters with racism or racial stress and trauma can cause physiological health outcomes ("weathering") that can lead to shorter life expectancy and chronic illness. Anti-Black gendered COVID-19 necropolitics brings together weathering and racial health disparities in a way that enables us to think through the deleterious intensification of pain and death during this moment for Black women, girls, and their families. The story of the bones of these girls, the death of Consuewella Africa, and the entire MOVE organization breathes new life into the struggle for justice, accountability, and reparations from the government and our educational institutions. Reflecting on the historical horrors of Philadelphia reminds us that the past is ever present. The fugitive breath of the bones of MOVE children coupled with the continued systematic murder of Black people and enduring racial traumas reveal the deep-rooted hatred of Black life.

I call for reparations as a response to anti-Black genocide using the United Nations (UN) definition of reparations. The UN developed five principles for reparations: restitution, which means restoring those harmed to the way they were prior to the harm; compensation, which means the perpetrating party provides financial redress for harm; rehabilitation, which provides legal, medical, psychological, and other services for those harmed; satisfaction, which brings repair for emotional, mental, or reputational injury; and, lastly, "guarantees of nonrepetition," which means stopping the harm and never repeating the injustice (UN General Assembly 2006, 7–8). Anything short of this basic five-pronged approach to reparations is inadequate. In 2015, the UN declared 2015 to 2024 as the International Decade for People of African Descent, to draw attention to the global marginalization, economic instability, state-sanctioned murder, health disparities, and other harms that Black people face due to the histories of transatlantic slavery, colonization, and systemic anti-Black racism (UN n.d.). This is why it was fitting when in 2021, the UN high commissioner for human rights, Michelle Bachelet, said, "I am calling on all states to stop denying—and start dismantling—racism; to end impunity and build trust; to listen to the voices of people of African descent; and to confront past legacies and deliver redress" (Associated Press 2021).

In her essay on mourning, Claudia Rankine illustrates the ways the movement for Black lives amounts to a movement for national mourning by forcing the public to recognize and lift up the lives of those murdered by the state (Rankine 2015). But what the treatment of the bones of MOVE children illustrated was that recognition is not enough. Reparations is the only adequate response to atone for Black death and the enduring harms caused to families. We have been taught to abstract Black death, to explain it away as singular rather than collective. We must be taught how to sit with the history of harm against Black people and with the reality of too many Black deaths, all the time: members of the MOVE family, Breonna Taylor, George Floyd, Ahmaud Arbery, Atatiana Jefferson, Bettie Jones, Botham Jean, India Kager, Sandra Bland, Michael Brown, Trayvon Martin, Dr. Susan Moore, and the others too numerous to name (Johnson 2020). Foregrounding ancestral breathing of those we have lost allows their bones to intuitively speak to us and inspire our collective breathing, healing, and restoration.

Abolishing Anti-Black COVID-19 Necropolitics with Fugitive Breath

This essay is an offering to Dr. Susan Moore, Consuewella Dotson Africa, Katricia "Tree" Africa, Zanetta Dotson Africa, and all those who have transitioned to become our ancestors. It is a living tribute to Chimére L. Smith, the MOVE family, Black women and girls living with long COVID, and all the Black families moving through trauma.

There is no cure. The only anecdote is an insistence upon breathing, an insistence upon freedom, and an insistence upon reparations by any and all means necessary.

For those of us left behind, still here carrying the weight of centuries of harm, carrying the torch for freedom, dancing in a new dawn at the intersection of slaveries' afterlives, fugitive breath guides us as we mourn. Under the dispensation of anti-Black gendered COVID-19 necropolitics, too many of us are uttering "I can't breathe" as our last words before we transition from the physical realm to the elsewhere. While our living as Black becomes prelude to death, how does sitting with death and still breathing become a fugitive act, a radical praxis that insists upon multiple realms of life? How can our insistence on breathing become tribute to ancestors we have gained and fortify us in the work for reparations and justice? What is breathing when anti-Blackness and COVID-19 are airborne viruses and wearing a mask is an act of political warfare rather than a health precaution? Breathing is a fugitive act. To be fugitive is to become clandestine, to eschew the will of law and societal mores sutured to the logic of Black death, and to insist upon living lives that matter. To consider Black lives valuable in a time of repetitious Black death, a death foretold before many of us were born, as Claudia Rankine writes, is an act of fugitivity. M. NourbeSe Philip reminds us that we must be breathed for before we can breathe, in order to live. We engage in fugitive breathing as a guide for surviving Black-corpse-lined logics of our current juridical, societal formation and the long-term harms and traumas of COVID-19. Fugitive breath means insisting on the full expansion of our lungs, despite the racist medical disinformation that Black lungs are somehow incapable of breathing properly (Braun 2014). Fugitive breath guides a refusal to accept the state-sanctioned project of anti-Black genocide through our witnessing and lifting up of our ancestors to breathe through us. The ancestral breath of our ancestors and all those who uttered "I can't breathe" is the breath that fortifies those of us who remain to witness, fight, and continue to move the needle toward justice.

Patrisse Cullors, the cofounder of the Black Lives Matter movement states that Black Lives Matter is "a spiritual movement. . . . Part of our calling as people who do this work for Black lives is to lift our people up, both in their living, but also in their death. . . . The need to lift our folks up feels so incredibly spirit-driven for me. . . . It is literally almost resurrecting a spirit so they can work through us to get the work that we need to get done" (Molina 2020). The notion of Black Lives Matter as a spiritual affirmation, a lifting up, a giving of breath, a resurrection in anti-Black space is an offering to honor our ancestors' continued work through us. We offer our breathing as a living tribute to engage in collective mourning, healing, and joy, to imagine and enact life-giving futures.

The dead animate our living as copresences—mediating, touching, influencing, and shaping our lives in a haunting that collapses time, makes the past present, and provides us with generational purpose. In her life-giving book, religious studies scholar Aisha Beliso-De Jesús reflects on the ways copresences center the religious practices of La Regla de Ocha (popularly known as Santería). She writes, "Copresences are Santería ontologies—they are the sensing of a multiplicity of being (and beings joined together) that are felt on the body, engaged with spiritually, experienced through television screens and divination, and expressed in diasporic assemblages. . . . Copresences are not simply dead or missing persons but rather are social figures of a past still present, proof that hauntings have taken place. They occupy the space of what we know to be true but cannot see" (2015, 9). Thinking about copresences with Beliso-De Jesús augments Cullors's discussion of Black Lives Matter working as spiritual affirmation that allows the dead to work through and with the living. Actively working with the dead provides a portal for thinking of the self not as singular but collective. The notion of thinking about the self in relation to or as part of the whole is rooted in I-n-I, or the Rastafari concept of oneness with the divine, which speaks to the mutual being of the physical and metaphysical realms (Bedasse 2017, 28). I-n-I suggests we are not simply individuals but exist in relation to others spiritually, physically, and environmentally. In this reading of I-n-I, the personal, as M. Jacqui Alexander (2005) writes, becomes the political and the spiritual. Interwoven in the political identities demarcating our lives by race, class, gender, sexuality, nationality etc., the spiritual realm becomes a copresent aspect of our identity that must be cared for. Functioning on a spiritual plane allows Black Lives Matter to engage multiple material and immaterial reservoirs to defend ourselves and assert a new vision for the world. Many thought the movement for Black lives was simply about the problem of policing, but the affirmation of Black life as valuable demands a dismantling of white supremacy and anti-Blackness that permeates all registers of society. It demands a real reckoning, which means an acknowledgement of harm, atonement, reparations, and a new world order premised on dignity, respect, justice, and freedom for all beings.

Rastafari, a Pan-African socio-spiritual movement, offers the concept of "transition" rather than death to illustrate that death is not a finality but an entrance to another form of being. Rastafari understands there is eternal life marked by a series of transitions from physical to metaphysical. In fact, a favorite Rastafari maxim is "We are spiritual beings having a human experience." The day of our birth marks the day we came to Earth in our human form, but we were alive long before we came to Earth and will live long after we are no longer housed in our physical temple. When death is discussed in normal parlance, finality or ending is considered, but when we look to Africana religions like La Regla de Ocha or Rastafari, we get a notion of copresent existences and eternal life, where the dead can animate the living, where we are our ancestors having a human experience, and where we continue the fight for reparations and dismantle all forms of oppression. M. NourbeSe Philip eloquently explains the relationship between the living and our ancestors in this way:

> When I invite the audience to read with me, we collectively engage in
> breathing for the Other—for those who
> couldn't breathe—then
> can't now
> and, perhaps, won't be able to.
> In doing so we give them a second life
> I can't breathe;
> I will breathe for you. (Philip 2018, 39)

Just as we were breathed for in the womb, we breathe for our ancestors throughout our lives. During this time of Black precarity globally, where the aggrieved rebel against necropower, racial capitalism, white supremacy, and genocide, it is important to reaffirm ways that Black people think about physical and metaphysical life by walking with ancestors. Black living in multiple mediums, seen and unseen, redacts the statistical glance at quantitative replays of Black death on the television by insisting on eternal Black life (Sharpe 2016).

Know that we will continue to breathe through the living once we transition to the spiritual realm. Our breath is not simply tied to mortality but to persistence and continuity of life. Our breath cyclically weaves in and between this world and the next in careful vibrational syncopation with Earth, with the ephemeral and the enduring. Our fugitive, irrational, chaotic breath claims life for us.

We become free as we commit our every breath to abolishing all forms of oppression. We become free through our mourning, our escape from death-worlds and creative conjuring of lifeworlds to come. Our insistence on using our fugitive breath, holding slow to our knowing, our inner center, is our plot to find a way through. If we live our lives as tribute, our breathing encompasses daily acts of defiance—we do not live only for ourselves. We live as though we have been here before, and it is only through the strength of our ancestors that we are able to dig deep to do the inner work necessary for our survival and the survival of our planet.

> Air . . . Breathe.
> Inhale . . . Exhale . . .
> Inhale . . . Exhale . . .
> Inhale . . . Exhale . . .
> Feel the air move in through your nostrils and out through your
>   slightly open lips.
> Deeply expand and contract your lungs. Feel the rise and fall of your
>   gentle life's breath.
> Cherish this breathing.
> In this moment.
> At this time.

Note

1. The term "fugitive breath" has been used by artist Julie Mehretu (2018) as part of the title for a drawing she made, but my conception of the term was not formed in consultation of her painting or another author. It is a term I am offering to describe my reflections during this time.

Bibliography

Adams, Dwight. 2021. "Dr. Susan Moore: What We Know About the Black Doctor Who Alleged Racism Before She Died." *Indianapolis Star*, May 12, 2021. https://www.indystar.com/story/news/health/2021/05/12/dr-susan-moore -what-we-know-black-doctor-who-alleged-racism/5056989001/.

Alexander, M. Jacqui. 2005. *Pedagogies of Crossing: Meditations on Feminism, Sexual Politics, Memory, and the Sacred.* Durham, NC: Duke University Press.

AMA (American Medical Association). 2021. *Organizational Strategic Plan to Embed Racial Justice and Advance Health Equity, 2021–2023.* Chicago:

American Medical Association. https://www.ama-assn.org/system/files/2021 -05/ama-equity-strategic-plan.pdf.

Associated Press. 2021. "The U.N. Rights Chief Says Reparations Are Needed for People Facing Racism," National Public Radio, June 28, 2021. https://www .npr.org/2021/06/28/1010870697/the-u-n-rights-chief-says-reparations-are -needed-for-people-facing-racism.

Bedasse, Monique. 2017. *Jah Kingdom: Rastafarians, Tanzania, and Pan-Africanism in the Age of Decolonization.* Chapel Hill: University of North Carolina Press.

Beliso-De Jesús, Aisha. 2015. *Electric Santería: Racial and Sexual Assemblages of Transnational Religion.* New York: Columbia University Press.

Braun, Lundy. 2014. *Breathing Race into the Machine: The Surprising Career of the Spirometer from Plantation to Genetics.* Minneapolis: University of Minnesota Press.

Burki, Talha. 2020. "Global Shortage of Personal Protective Equipment." *Lancet Infectious Diseases* 20 no. 7 (July): 785–86. https://doi.org/10.1016%2FS1473 -3099(20)30501-6.

CDC (Centers for Disease Control and Prevention). 2020a. "Risk for COVID-19 Infection, Hospitalization, and Death By Race/Ethnicity." National Center for Immunization and Respiratory Diseases. Updated July 28, 2022. https:// www.cdc.gov/coronavirus/2019-ncov/covid-data/investigations-discovery /hospitalization-death-by-race-ethnicity.html.

———. 2020b. "Health Equity Considerations and Racial and Ethnic Minority Groups." National Center for Immunization and Respiratory Diseases. Updated July 24, 2020. https://stacks.cdc.gov/view/cdc/91049.

Chinnappan, Shivani. 2021. "Long COVID: The Impact on Women and Ongoing Research." Society for Women's Health Research, March 18, 2021. https:// swhr.org/long-covid-the-impact-on-women-and-ongoing-research/.

Collins, Francis S. 2021. "NIH Launches New Initiative to Study 'Long COVID.'" National Institutes of Health, February 23, 2021. https://www.nih.gov/about -nih/who-we-are/nih-director/statements/nih-launches-new-initiative -study-long-covid.

Cooney, Elizabeth. 2021. "Researchers Fear People of Color May Be Disproportionately Affected by Long Covid." STAT, May 10, 2021. https://www.stat news.com/2021/05/10/with-long-covid-history-may-be-repeating-itself -among-people-of-color/.

Davies, Dave. 2020. "Reckoning with the Dead: Journalist Goes Inside an NYC COVID-19 Disaster Morgue." National Public Radio, May 28, 2020.

https://www.npr.org/sections/health-shots/2020/05/28/863710050/reckoning -with-the-dead-journalist-goes-inside-an-nyc-covid-19-disaster-morgue.

Demby, Gene, host. 2018. "Making the Case That Discrimination Is Bad for Your Health." *Codeswitch Podcast.* January 14, 2018. https://www.npr.org /sections/codeswitch/2018/01/14/577664626/making-the-case-that-discrim ination-is-bad-for-your-health.

Democracy Now! 2020. "'This Is How Black People Get Killed': Dr. Susan Moore Dies of COVID After Decrying Racist Care." December 30, 2020. https://www.democracynow.org/2020/12/30/dr_susan_moore_healthcare _racism.

dos Santos, Hebert Luan Pereira Campos, Fernanda Beatriz Melo Maciel, Kênia Rocha Santos, Cídia Dayara Vieira Silva da Conceição, Rian Silva de Oliveira, Natiene Ramos Ferreira da Silva, and Nília Maria de Brito Lima Prado. 2020. "Necropolitics and the Impact of COVID-19 on the Black Community in Brazil: A Literature Review and a Document Analysis." *Ciência and Saúde Coletiva* 25, supplement 2 (October): 4211–24. https://doi.org/10.1590/1413 -812320202510.2.25482020.

Ducharme, Jamie. 2021. "Black Women Are Fighting to Be Recognized as Long Covid Patients." *Time*, April 12, 2021. https://time.com/5954132/black -women-long-covid/.

Eligon, John. 2020. "Black Doctor Dies of Covid-19 After Complaining of Racist Treatment." *New York Times*, December 23, 2020. https://www.nytimes.com /2020/12/23/us/susan-moore-black-doctor-indiana.html.

Fadulu, Lola. 2022. "Experts Warn of Racial Disparities in the Diagnosis and Treatment of Long Covid." *New York Times*, March 29, 2022. https://www .nytimes.com/2022/03/29/health/long-covid-black.html

Fanon, Frantz. 2008. *Black Skin, White Masks.* London: Pluto.

Flaherty, Colleen. 2021a. "A Mystery and a Scandal for Anthropology." *Inside Higher Ed*, April 23, 2021. https://www.insidehighered.com/news/2021/04 /23/anthropological-mystery-involving-penn-and-princeton-scandal-too.

———. 2021b. "Penn, Princeton Apologize for Treatment of MOVE Bombing Victim's Remains." *Inside Higher Ed*, April 29, 2021. https://www.inside highered.com/quicktakes/2021/04/29/penn-princeton-apologize-treatment -move-bombing-victims-remains.

Geronimus, Arline T., Margaret Hicken, Danya Keene, and John Bound. 2006. "'Weathering' and Age Patterns of Allostatic Load Scores Among Blacks and Whites in the United States." *American Journal of Public Health* 96, no. 5 (May): 826–33. https://doi.org/10.2105/AJPH.2004.060749.

Goodin-Smith, Oona, and Mensah M. Dean. 2021. "Consuewella Dotson Africa, Longtime MOVE Member, Dies at 67." *Philadelphia Inquirer*, June 16, 2021. https://www.inquirer.com/obituaries/consuewella-dotson-africa-dead-move-philadelphia-20210616.html.

Gravlee, Clarence. 2020. "Racism, Not Genetics, Explains Why Black Americans Are Dying of COVID-19." *Scientific American*, June 7, 2020. https://blogs.scientificamerican.com/voices/racism-not-genetics-explains-why-black-americans-are-dying-of-covid-19/.

Health Justice Commons. n.d. "Terms Defined: Medical Industrial Complex (MIC)." Accessed August 9, 2022. https://www.healthjusticecommons.org/terms-defined.

Johnson, L. A. 2020. "A Decade of Watching Black People Die." National Public Radio, May 31, 2020. https://www.npr.org/2020/05/29/865261916/a-decade-of-watching-black-people-die.

Kassutto, Maya. 2021. "Remains of Children Killed in MOVE Bombing Sat in a Box at Penn Museum for Decades." Billy Penn, April 21, 2021. https://billypenn.com/2021/04/21/move-bombing-penn-museum-bones-remains-princeton-africa/?utm_source=dlvr.itandutm_medium=twitter.

Lanziotti, Vanessa S., Yonca Bulut, Danilo Buonsenso, and Sebastion Gonzalez-Dambrauskas. 2022. "Vaccine Apartheid: This Is Not the Way to End the Pandemic." *Journal of Pediatrics and Child Health* 58, no. 2 (February): 228–31. https://doi.org/10.1111/jpc.15805.

Mack, Justin L. 2020. "Dr. Susan Moore: What We Know About the Black Doctor's Claims of Racism at Carmel Hospital." *Indianapolis Star*, December 29, 2020. https://www.indystar.com/story/news/local/indianapolis/2020/12/29/dr-susan-moore-indiana-what-we-know-her-life-and-death/4071090001/.

Mast, Jason. 2014. "'We Charge Genocide' Issues Damning Report on Abuse and Brutality in Chicago." Juvenile Justice Information Exchange, October 24, 2014. https://jjie.org/2014/10/24/we-charge-genocide-issues-damning-report-on-abuse-and-brutality-in-chicago/.

Mayo Clinic Staff. 2022. "COVID-19: Long-Term Effects." Mayo Clinic. June 28, 2022. https://www.mayoclinic.org/diseases-conditions/coronavirus/in-depth/coronavirus-long-term-effects/art-20490351#.

Mbembe, Achille. 2003. "Necropolitics." *Public Culture* 15, no. 1 (Winter): 11–40. https://doi.org/10.1080/17441692.2021.1906927.

McCrystal, Laura. 2020. "Philly City Council Has Formally Apologized for the Deadly 1985 MOVE Bombing." *Philadelphia Inquirer*, Nov 16, 2020. https://www.inquirer.com/news/philadelphia/move-bombing-apology-philadelphia-walter-wallace-20201112.html.

Mehretu, Julie. 2018. *Fugitive Breath Drawing*. Ink and acrylic on paper, 26 1/8 × 40". Marian Goodman Gallery, New York.

Messerschmidt, James W. 2021. "Donald Trump, Dominating Masculine Necropolitics, and COVID-19." *Men and Masculinities* 24, no. 1 (April): 189–94. https://doi.org/10.1177%2F1097184X20984816.

Molina, Alejandra. 2020. "Black Lives Matter Is 'a Spiritual Movement,' Says Co-Founder Patrisse Cullors." Religion News Service, June 15, 2020. https://religionnews.com/2020/06/15/why-black-lives-matter-is-a-spiritual-movement-says-blm-co-founder-patrisse-cullors/.

Philip, M. NourbeSe. "The Ga(s)p." 2018. In *Poetics and Precarity*, edited by Myung Mi Kim and Christanne Miller, 31–40. Albany: State University of New York Press.

Rankine, Claudia. 2015. "The Condition of Black Life Is One of Mourning." *New York Times Magazine*, June 22, 2015. https://www.nytimes.com/2015/06/22/magazine/the-condition-of-black-life-is-one-of-mourning.html.

Richardson, Rashida. 2020. "Government Data Practices as Necropolitics and Racial Arithmetic." Global Data Justice, October 8, 2020. https://globaldatajustice.org/covid-19/necropolitics-racial-arithmetic.

Roane, J. T. 2021. "The Shocking MOVE Bombing Was Part of a Broader Pattern of Anti-Black Racism." *Washington Post*, May 13, 2021. https://www.washingtonpost.com/outlook/2021/05/13/shocking-move-bombing-was-part-broader-pattern-anti-black-racism/.

Roberts, Sam. "Consuewella Africa, 67, Dies; Lost Two Daughters in MOVE Siege." *New York Times*, June 21, 2021. https://www.nytimes.com/2021/06/21/us/consuewella-africa-dead.html?searchResultPosition=7.

Rubin, Rita. 2020. "As Their Numbers Grow, COVID-19 'Long Haulers' Stump Experts." *Journal of the American Medical Association* 324, no. 14: 1381–83. https://doi.org/10.1001/jama.2020.17709.

Rudavsky, Shari. 2021. "Here's What IU Health Investigation Says About Death of Dr. Susan Moore Who Alleged Racism." *Indianapolis Star*, May 12, 2021. https://www.indystar.com/story/news/health/2021/05/12/dr-susan-moore-iu-health-releases-report-death-black-doctor/5044308001/.

Rushovich, Tamara, and Sarah S. Richardson. 2021. "The Intersection of Black Women, COVID, and Death Rates." *Boston Globe*, April 5, 2021. https://www.bostonglobe.com/2021/04/05/opinion/black-women-are-dying-covid-19-higher-rates-than-almost-every-other-group/?event=event12.

Sandset, Tony. 2021. "The Necropolitics of COVID-19: Race, Class and Slow Death in an Ongoing Pandemic." *Global Public Health* 16, no. 8–9: 1411–23. https://doi.org/10.1080/17441692.2021.1906927.

Select Subcommittee on the Coronavirus Crisis. 2021. "New GAO Report Details Trump Administration's Failed Coronavirus Response." January 28, 2021. https://coronavirus.house.gov/news/press-releases/new-gao-report -details-trump-administration-s-failed-coronavirus-response.

Shaban, Hamza. 2014. "How Racism Creeps into Medicine: The History of a Medical Instrument Reveals the Dubious Science of Racial Difference." *Atlantic*, August 29, 2014. https://www.theatlantic.com/health/archive/2014/08 /how-racism-creeps-into-medicine/378618/.

Sharpe, Christina. 2016. *In the Wake: On Blackness and Being*. Durham, NC: Duke University Press.

Siegel, Zachary A., Abigail Brown, Andrew Devendorf, Johanna Collier, and Leonard A. Jason 2018. "A Content Analysis of Chronic Fatigue Syndrome and Myalgic Encephalomyelitis in the News from 1987 to 2013." *Chronic Illness* 14, no. 1 (March): 3–12. https://doi.org/10.1177/1742395317703175.

Sitz, Lindsey. 2021. "Why This Black Woman with 'Long Covid' Feels the Medical Community Has Failed Her." *Washington Post*, February 2, 2021. https:// www.washingtonpost.com/video/topics/coronavirus/why-this-black-woman -with-long-covid-feels-the-medical-community-has-failed-her/2021/02/02 /68ce212c-f1ba-4983-8d07-d2fd5e8e4429_video.html.

Smith, Chimére L. 2021. "Congressional Testimony from Patient-Led Advocate Chimére L. Smith." The You + ME Registry + Biobank, May 25, 2021. https://youandmeregistry.com/congressional-testimony-from-patient-led -advocate-chimere-l-smith/.

———. n.d. "About." Accessed July 5, 2022. https://chimereladawn.com/about.

Smith, Christen. 2016. "Facing the Dragon: Black Mothering, Sequelae, and Gendered Necropolitics in the Americas." *Transforming Anthropology* 24, no. 1 (April): 31–48. https://doi.org/10.1111/traa.12055.

Sudre, Carole H., Benjamine Murray, Thomas Varsavsky, Mark S. Graham, Rose S. Penfold, Ruth C. Bowyer, Joan Capdevila Pujol, et al. 2021. "Attributes and Predictors of Long COVID." *Nature Medicine* 27: 626–31. https://doi.org/10 .1038/s41591-021-01292-y.

Thompson, Alison E., Benjamin L. Ranard, Ying Wei, and Sanja Jelic. 2020. "Prone Positioning in Awake, Nonintubated Patients with COVID-19 Hypoxemic Respiratory Failure." *Journal of American Medical Association Internal Medicine* 180, no. 11: 1537–39. https://doi.org/10.1001/jamainternmed .2020.3030.

UN (United Nations). n.d. "International Decade for People of African Descent 2015–2024." https://www.un.org/en/observances/decade-people-african -descent/background.

UN General Assembly. 2006. Basic Principles and Guidelines on the Right to a Remedy and Reparation for Victims of Gross Violations of International Human Rights Law and Serious Violations of International Humanitarian Law. Resolution adopted by the General Assembly on March 21, 2006. https://www.un.org/ruleoflaw/files/BASICP~1.PDF.

U.S. Government Accountability Office. 2021. "COVID-19: Critical Vaccine Distribution, Supply Chain, Program Integrity, and Other Challenges Require Focused Federal Attention." January 28, 2021. https://www.gao.gov/products /gao-21-265.

Weber, Paul J., and Sarah Rankin. 2020. "Overwhelmed with COVID-19 Cases, Hospital Start Converting Chapels, Cafeterias, Parking Garages: 'We're in Trouble.'" *Chicago Tribune*, November 18, 2020. https://www.chicagotribune .com/coronavirus/ct-nw-coronavirus-cases-hospitals-20201118-4zm3lth mvnb4xm53yggqwnh2gu-story.html.

Our Ethic of Care

On Doing Black Feminist Work When You Listen to the Ancestors

Julia S. Jordan-Zachery

Dear [Name]

Thank you for your abstract proposal. Based on your proposal [title], I would like to invite you to submit to the volume "Black Women and da 'Rona: Community, Consciousness, and Ethics of Care." This invitation does not guarantee that your submission will be included in the book. After submission, it will go through an initial review.

As part of compiling this edited volume, I offer this ethic of care. I want to center the humanity of Black femmes, girls, and women in this writing and, as such, was compelled to think through how to approach this project critically.

Working in Community

In part, I came to this project because Black women often heal in community. To honor that, I thought it would be important to organize small writing groups consisting of three authors (or three teams). Much of the academy is set up around individualism. As a way of countering this, I'm willing to help organize small writing/ working groups. You have to opt into this by emailing me (July 3, 2020). These writing groups are designed to help you sustain your project.

Time of Submission

Your submission is due on/or before November 13, 2020, at 4 p.m. EST. Please communicate with me if you need to deviate from this time frame. The goal is to have a solid working project by January 2021. This means that I will conduct an initial review and, if needed, engage with you about ways to strengthen your submission. Once you receive my response, you will have three weeks to engage any edits, etc., and return the submission. My goal is to foster open and engaged communication with you. But I can't do it alone. So, I ask you to please be in dialogue with me as this project unfolds.

Submission Checklist

The Cover Page

___ Title

___ Name

___ Contact Information

___ Abstract (150–200 words)

Engaging Our Stories About Black Women

As we write, I want us to think carefully and critically about how we describe and offer details on Black femmes, girls, and women. Language matters. So, for example, are you using a language that suggests that Black femmes, girls, and women are broken and in need of fixing? In this volume, we want to tell the truth about Black femmes, girls, and women, *and* we also want to be mindful of not perpetuating existing narratives and tropes.

___ I am mindful of not perpetuating existing harmful narratives and tropes.

Black as a Racial Group

____ I capitalized Black when referring to the racial group.

Conscientious Engagement with Literature (primarily for those working on academic/scholarly papers)

____ I cited Black women. Please cite Black women!

____ I actively engaged with the scholarship of Black women and not simply just referenced their name.

____ I cited a junior faculty member.

____ I cited myself, if appropriate.

____ I moved beyond the canon to include at least one "fresh" name.

Note on Proofreading

____ Have I proofread my submission?

Suggestions on how to proofread

a. Have someone read it for you.

b. Read the last sentence first and work backward.

c. Read it out loud.

d. Record it as you read and then listen to it—a few days later.

e. Give yourself time to think, write, and then edit.

____ I accepted changes.

____ I turned off Track Changes.

____ I used Times New Roman, 12-point font.

____ I followed the formatting of the Chicago Manual of Style (for those writing academic/scholarly papers).

____ I have page numbers, and they are positioned in the top right corner.

____ I spelled out acronyms the first time I used them.

____ I checked for passive voice. A corny, but a good way to check for passive voice—use "by zombies" (see the National Archives' guide "Passive Voice and Zombies," https://www.archives.gov /open/plain-writing/tips/passive-voice.html).

___ Did I overuse -ly words? Often words ending in -ly are not needed. So, do the -ly check and delete where necessary.

___ Did I double-space?

___ I wrote no more than 20 pages, double spaced, and including references (for those writing academic/scholarly papers).

___ I wrote no more than 2,500 words, double spaced (for those writing prose/poetry, etc.).

___ I spell checked and checked the vocabulary.

Citations (for those writing academic/scholarly papers)

___ I used the Chicago Manual of Style.

___ I cited myself.

___ All citations follow the in-text method (no use of footnotes/endnotes for citations).

___ All endnotes/footnotes are placed at the end of the document.

The Nitty-Gritty of Writing

___ I wrote my introduction last to ensure that it truly captures what I'm writing about.

___ My title fits well with my chapter. It is short and to the point.

___ I highlighted, in the introduction, what this chapter is about. Is it easily identifiable?

___ I explained to the reader why this paper is important, what gap it is filling, and what its central contribution is, and it is all easily identifiable in the introduction.

___ I did not just end the paper; I have a substantive conclusion.

___ I checked to determine that I have topic sentences in each paragraph.

___ I checked my transitions between and within paragraphs.

___ Jargon, I minimized my use of jargon.

___ I wrote in an accessible manner for folks outside of my discipline or even the academy.

____ I wrote in a manner that is clear, concise, and to the point.

____ My submission fits the call for chapters.

Methods, Data, Tables, Figures, Images, and Appendices

____ I have clearly and succinctly articulated how I'm doing what I'm
doing. That is, my method/approach is clearly articulated and
can be followed by others outside of the discipline.

____ I have concisely shown who is involved or what is involved to
help me make my argument. My data is clear.

____ My tables and figures are referenced and explained in text and
are clearly labeled.

____ All images are referenced and explained in the text, and the
image is clearly and visibly replicated in the submission.

____ I've attached my appendices.

Permissions Are Key

____ I have permission to cite/reuse previously published works. I
have included this along with my submission.

____ IRB permission, do I need it? I include evidence that I have it.

Original Submission

____ I am sure that this is an original submission and that it is not
currently published or under review with another entity.

In Community, We Submit This Project Together

____ I have recommended at least one reviewer of this edited volume.

Submission

____ I submitted my chapter as a Word document!

Congratulations. Now let's celebrate what we have created together.

CONTRIBUTORS

Dr. Shamara Wyllie Alhassan is an assistant professor of religious studies with a focus on the Black experience in the Americas in the School of Historical, Philosophical and Religious Studies at Arizona State University. Alhassan specializes in Africana women's radical epistemologies. Her forthcoming manuscript, "Re-Membering the Maternal Goddess: Rastafari Women's Intellectual History and Activism in the Pan-African World," is the winner of the 2019 National Women's Association and the University of Illinois Press First Book Prize.

Dr. Sharnnia Artis is the assistant dean of access and inclusion for the Henry Samueli School of Engineering and Donald Bren School of Information and Computer Sciences at the University of California, Irvine (UCI). She is responsible for programs at the pre-college, undergraduate, and graduate levels to facilitate the recruitment, retention, and overall success of students from traditionally underrepresented groups in engineering and information and computer sciences. Dr. Artis has over eighteen years of experience working with education and outreach programs in engineering and has authored over thirty-five publications in STEM education and outreach. Prior to joining UCI, she was the education and outreach director for the Center for Energy Efficient Electronics Science at the University of California, Berkeley. Previously, Dr. Artis spent nine years at Virginia

Tech, providing program and student support for the Center for the Enhancement of Engineering Diversity, and she has four years of industry and government experience as a human factors engineer. Dr. Artis holds a BS, MS, and PhD in industrial and systems engineering from Virginia Tech.

Dr. Keisha L. Bentley-Edwards is the associate director of research for the Samuel DuBois Cook Center on Social Equity and an associate professor at Duke University's School of Medicine. Dr. Bentley-Edwards's research focuses on how racism, gender, and culture influence development throughout the life span, especially for African Americans. Her research emphasizes cultural strengths and eliminating structural barriers to support health development in communities, families, and students. Dr. Bentley-Edwards has published and lectured extensively on the use of racial socialization and racial cohesion strategies to facilitate positive outcomes for high school and college students. She is dedicated to eliminating barriers to healthy birth and pregnancy outcomes. Dr. Bentley-Edwards nurtures complex conversations around race and racism in ways that not only identify disparities but prompt meaningful strategies for remedying these disparities. Her research has been supported by the Robert Wood Johnson Foundation and the National Institutes of Health. Dr. Bentley-Edwards regularly shares her expertise on the role of structural racism and bias on health, education, and social outcomes with families, policy makers, practitioners, and the media, including the *New York Times*, *USA Today*, the *Washington Post*, and *CBS News*.

Dr. Candace S. Brown is an assistant professor of gerontology in the Department of Public Health Sciences at University of North Carolina at Charlotte and a research collaborator with the Motivated Cognition and Aging Brain Lab at Duke University. As a former K–5 health teacher, her interdisciplinary research and teaching focus is on understanding the psychosocial and neurological exercise motivations of the life course with a focus on older adults. Her most recent work has been published in *Gerontology and Geriatrics Education*, *Women's Health Reports*, and *Sports*. She is the mother of three busy kids, ages fifteen, fourteen, and twelve.

Jenny Douglas is a senior lecturer in health promotion at the Open University and the chair and founder of the Black Women's Health and Wellbeing Research Network.

Kaja Dunn is an assistant professor of theatre and teaches acting at the University of North Carolina at Charlotte, and works as an actor, director, and intimacy choreographer with Theatrical Intimacy Education. She has presented her work on training theatre students of color at Goldsmiths, University of London; Southeastern Theatre Conference (SETC) and SETC Theatre Symposium; Kennedy Center American College Theater Festival; and the Association for Theatre in Higher Education, among other places. She is the secretary of the Black Theatre Association. She has taught and performed internationally. Kaja was previously a lecturer at California State University San Marcos and toured with Ya Tong Theatre in Taiwan. Her primary research focus is on culturally competent practices in theatre and theatre training. Other teaching credits include working with homeless and foster youth with Playwrights Project in San Diego and as a teaching artist with Young Audiences. She is the mother of three smart, energetic boys, ages three, six, and ten.

Onisha Etkins (ID: Onisha, she, her, hers) learned what love, agency, and power looked like through the movement and dance of her family members. Family limin' and winin' sessions taught her how liberation and movement through dance are one and the same. Raised by two Guyanese parents in Brooklyn, New York, her understanding of community resilience was formed by the beautiful West Indian neighborhood she grew up in. She received her bachelor's degree in science, technology, and society and her master of science degree in community health and prevention research from Stanford University, and she is currently pursuing a PhD in population health sciences at the Harvard T. H. Chan School of Public Health. She is passionate about the mental health of people(s) across the Caribbean Diaspora and is particularly interested in how dance and music have been, and continue to be, sites of pleasure and bodily understanding for Caribbean communities. She describes herself as a part-time PhD student and full-time dancehall/soca dancer and Carnivalist. You can catch her talking about how she navigates all of her passions and academia on her YouTube channel as Dr. Rude Gyal.

Rhonda M. Gonzales is a professor of African and African Diaspora history at the University of Texas at San Antonio. Her research combines the use of comparative linguistics, ethnography, oral tradition, and more to recover early history. Sample publications include "Historical Linguistics: Words and Things" in the Oxford Research Encyclopedia of African History and *Societies, Religion, and History: Central-East Tanzanians and the World They Created, c. 200 BCE to 1800 CE* published by Columbia University Press. Co-authored publications include *Bantu Africa: 3500 BCE to Present*, "Gender, Authority, and Identity in African History: Heterarchy, Cosmic Families, and Lifestages" in *The Palgrave Handbook of African Women's Studies*, and a book forthcoming with Cambridge University Press, *Family Before Gender: History in Central and Eastern Africa, ca. 500–1900.*

Endia Hayes is a doctoral student at Rutgers University in the Department of Sociology. She studies formerly enslaved Afro-Texan women and how they engage with storytelling, land, and the archive to form radical ways of knowing. Endia's work frames enslaved women as social theorists who have reimagined Texas culture and history.

Ashley E. Hollingshead is a doctoral student of sociology at Rutgers University. Her work focuses on Black women's experiences with policing and surveillance in gentrified communities. Ashley mentors young Black women and men on character development, lifting while she climbs.

Dr. Kendra Jason is an assistant professor of sociology at the University of North Carolina at Charlotte. She is an interdisciplinary health disparities scholar who examines the links between race, discrimination, work engagement, and care processes for older Black adults. She has most recently published in outlets such as the *Gerontologist, Journal of Applied Gerontology, Health Care Management Review,* and *Research in the Sociology of Work,* and her work has been featured on Forbes.com. She is the parent of one cool eleven-year-old kid.

Dr. Julia S. Jordan-Zachery is a professor in and chair of the Women's, Gender, and Sexuality Studies Department at Wake Forest University. She has written a number of articles and several books, including the award-winning *Black Women, Cultural Images and Social Policy,* and she is the co-editor of *Black Girl Magic Beyond the Hashtag: Twenty-First-Century Acts of Self-Definition* and the editor of *Lavender Fields: Black Women Experiencing Fear, Agency, and Hope in the Time of COVID-19.* She has also produced the documentary *Healing Roots* and a poetry book, *Eat the Meat and Spit Out the Bones.*

Dr. Stacie LeSure is the founder and CEO of Engineers for Equity (E4E). E4E is a socially conscious organization committed to applying evidence-based professional development strategies to inspire current and future STEM professionals to become more self-aware, empathetic, and emotionally intelligent. She earned a PhD in engineering education at Utah State University. She also has a master of science in materials science and engineering from Georgia Institute of Technology and a bachelor of science in physics from Spelman College. Dr. LeSure's current research interests focus on inclusive pedagogical practices as well as the integration of human-centered design and service learning opportunities to recruit and retain students in engineering degree programs.

Dr. Janaka B. Lewis is the director of the Women's and Gender Studies Program, an associate professor of English, and a faculty affiliate in the Department of Africana Studies at the University of North Carolina at Charlotte. She is the author of *Freedom Narratives of African American Women* and has contributed essays and chapters on race and gender dynamics in higher education. She is the author of two children's books, *Brown All Over* and *Bold Nia Marie Passes the Test* that she has shared in research and presentations on diversity in children's literature, and she is currently working on a monograph about Black girlhood and narratives of play in literature and media. She is the parent of two children, ages nine and six.

Dr. Michelle Meggs is the executive director of the Women + Girls Research Alliance at the University of North Carolina at Charlotte. She holds a doctorate of arts in humanities with a focus on Africana women's studies from Clark Atlanta University and a master of divinity degree from Wake Forest University. As an activist scholar, her research interests focus on interrogating and deconstructing negative images of Black women in popular culture, building empowering narratives around Black women's lives, and affirming the strengths of Black girlhood and womanhood. She is a sought-after workshop speaker on women's empowerment, leadership, and embracing ratchetness as a form of liberation.

Nitya Mehrotra is an undergraduate student at the University of California, Irvine, studying biological sciences. Her research interests include the mental health struggles and coping mechanisms utilized by Black women in computer science and engineering graduate programs, as well as comparing students who attended predominantly white institutions for undergraduate programs versus those who attended historically Black colleges and universities.

Sherine Andreine Powerful (ID: Sherine, Mx., she, they) is a dedicated daughter of the Caribbean sand, sun, and sea, having been born in Kingston, Jamaica; spending the formative years of her childhood in a West Indian neighborhood in the Boogie Down Bronx; and contributing to the region through advocacy and public health work in different CARICOM (Caribbean Community and Common Market) countries. She received her bachelor's degree in Latin American studies (Caribbean concentration) and international studies from Yale University and holds a master of public health degree in population and family health, with a concentration in global health, from the Columbia University Mailman School of Public Health. As a doctor of public health (DrPH) student at the Harvard T. H. Chan School of Public Health, her interests are centered around the English-speaking Caribbean and include feminist global health and development leadership; gender and sexual health, equity, and justice; pleasure, healing, and liberation; and resilience and anti-colonial sustainable development in the context of climate change. If you can catch her, you'll probably find her obsessing over the color turquoise, bussin' a "shake and a jiggle and a bubble and a dip," or scheming on her next Carnival/Masquerade/J'ouvert adventures!

Dr. Marjorie Shavers is an associate professor and the department head of Counseling, Leadership and Special Education at Missouri State University. She has a PhD in counselor education from the Ohio

State University and is currently licensed as a professional school and professional clinical counselor with supervision designation. Dr. Shavers's research agenda focuses on exploring how educational systems and professionals impact the experiences and overall mental health of students, particularly Black women. Dr. Shavers's most recent work focuses specifically on the experiences of Black women pursuing doctorate and postdoctorate degrees in computer science and engineering. In addition to her research, her teaching and clinical practice is aimed at enhancing mental health among Black women. Dr. Shavers was recognized as the 2015 Counselor Educator of the Year from the Ohio Association of Counselor Education and Supervision and received the Distinguished Research and Scholarship Award at Heidelberg University.

Breauna Marie Spencer is a doctoral candidate at the University of California, Irvine (UCI), in the Department of Sociology. She also received her undergraduate degrees in sociology and education sciences and master's degrees in demographic and social analysis and sociology at UCI. Ms. Spencer is also a lecturer at Loyola Marymount University. Overall, her research interests include examining the academic, social, and psychological experiences of women and racially underrepresented students within engineering and computer science degree programs at both the undergraduate and graduate level. Ms. Spencer's research has been published in *Sociological Forum* and *Fat Studies*, among other outlets.

Dr. Tehia Starker Glass is the Cato College of Education director of diversity and inclusion and an associate professor of elementary education and educational psychology at University of North Carolina at Charlotte. Her research and publications focus on preparing preservice and in-service teachers' culturally responsive teaching self-efficacy, anti-racism curriculum development, culturally responsive classroom management, and exploring how caregivers and teachers discuss race with children. Dr. Glass works with teachers, schools, and districts around the country to revise their instruction and curriculum to be more anti-racism oriented. Dr. Glass is currently working on her academic book and a children's book to assist caregivers and teachers to have conversations about race with children. She codesigned and is the program director of a four-course Anti-Racism in Urban Education Graduate Certificate Program. Her commentary on anti-racism has been included on CNN.com.

Amber Walker earned a master of history from the University of Texas at San Antonio. Walker's research focus is early East African history, migration, and refugee studies, and she has completed field research on Somali Bantu migration and Chinese migration to Tanzania. Walker currently teaches Advanced Placement U.S. History at YES Prep Public Schools in Houston, Texas.

INDEX